HOLDING IT ALL TOGETHER WHEN YOU'RE HYPERMOBILE

CHRISTIE COX

Holding It All Together When You're Hypermobile

ISBN: 979-8-9861264-0-1 (Print)
ISBN: 979-8-9861264-1-8 (ebook)

TABLE OF CONTENTS

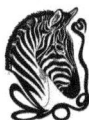

DEDICATION

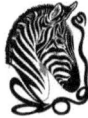

To my joyous, unwavering loving and supportive husband, John. He loves me like no one else ever has and ever will. Without his ongoing support, I would not be here. He joins me in the hope that the hard-fought lessons, knowledge, and our personal experiences can help others better cope and their loved ones better understand.

DISCLAIMER

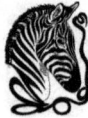

This book details the author's personal experiences with and opinions about managing chronic pain and illness with coexisting physical and psychological disorders. The author and publisher are providing this book and its contents on an "as is" basis and make no representations or warranties of any kind with respect to this book or its contents. The author and publisher disclaim all such representations and warranties, including, for example, warranties of merchantability and health care for a particular purpose. In addition, the author and publisher do not represent or warrant that the information accessible via this book is accurate, complete, or current. The statements made about products and services have not been evaluated by the US Food and Drug Administration. They are not intended to diagnose, treat, cure, or prevent any condition or disease. Please consult with your own physician or licensed health care specialist regarding the suggestions and recommendations made in this book. Except as specifically stated in this book, neither the author or publisher nor any authors, contributors, or other representatives will be liable for damages arising out of or in connection with the use of this book. This is a comprehensive limitation of liability that applies to all damages of any kind, including (without limitation) compensatory; direct, indirect, or consequential damages; loss of data, income, or profit; and loss of or damage to property and claims of third parties. You understand that this book is not intended as a substitute for seeing a health care practitioner. Before you begin any health care program or change your lifestyle in any way, it is imperative that you consult your physician, a licensed mental health provider, or other licensed health care practitioner to ensure that you are in good health and that the examples contained in this book will not harm you. Use of this book implies your acceptance of this disclaimer.

STRAIGHT FROM THE ZEBRA'S MOUTH

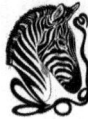

In life, we encounter many dark nights of the soul, wherein the intensity of the moment, life can feel completely hopeless. But if we hold on until the next day things can change. An incremental shift in our thinking, a gradual acceptance, or a sudden change in our circumstances can radically alter how we view our situation from one day to the next. "It won't always feel like this" is a mantra that always rings true no matter what situation we're in or where we are in our life's journey.

– Linzi Clark

Let's start by establishing the end goal right up front — to be better. That is the goal. Is it achievable when you have a chronic illness? I believe it is.

Dr. Wayne W. Dyer used to say in his speeches, "Your goal isn't to be better than anyone else. Your goal is to be better than you used to be." That quote has always resonated with me. If you set the goal of being better than you used to be, then you're succeeding in your own life journey. We're all on different life paths, so the improvements that I needed to make may not be the same as those you need (and vice versa).

The purpose of this book is to help *you* understand how you might be able to change *your* circumstances by changing your habits, actions, and behaviors to enhance *your* life experience. My suggestions, resources, and tools are things I have done with success. They boil down to a set of simple ways to improve your overall well-being through the practice of daily, practical, and healthy habits.

This book is written to help anyone who is chronically ill with hypermobile Ehlers-Danlos syndrome (hEDS), searching for answers and cannot obtain the correct diagnosis, the right doctor to help, or the treatment for life-long (and sometimes rare) medical conditions that have no answers. But it is also written to honor your journey and let you know you are seen and heard. I understand and can empathize because I have been there. This book is meant to help you feel validated for all the struggles you are facing.

I have pulled from various resources, my own experiences, fellow patients, and online public forums to collectively gather this list of healing habits. I am not a medical provider and have no medical training, and I can only share my limited personal experience. I recognize EDS manifests itself in various ways for different people, so I do not expect all of the suggestions to help everyone. But I do believe that there are more than just a few nuggets of helpful information for you or someone you care about who might be dealing with hEDS. I want to share with you what I learned over the last decade so that you can avoid some of the mistakes that I made and live a more fulfilling life.

One thing is incontrovertibly true for people with a chronic disease: If you don't make time for your wellness, you'll later be forced to make time for your illness. This book isn't just about getting over being sick. It's also about warding off disease by working through work-life balance challenges, reprioritizing your life, tackling today's demanding lifestyle through effective stress management, and learning important lessons on actually being present and choosing joy and happiness in your life despite illness.

Why you should read this book

Tired of being told there's no name or treatment for your illness? That you're just making it up for attention? That your pain is imaginary or that it can't be real because you're too young/old/pretty/bright/healthy/normal to have a chronic disorder?

You are not alone! I know because I've been there. Prior to my diagnosis, my life used to be unmanageable, and there have been times since that I've still felt alone, confused, frustrated, and even hopeless. I understand the chronic pain and fatigue and feelings of being dismissed by medical professionals and loved ones alike. It is like pushing a boulder uphill sometimes when your body gives out just as you think you are getting stronger again. But slowly I've worked my way back to health and happiness and discovered on the way that the process I took to find my way back could help others. There are techniques that can help you self-manage the flares and hope to live well with hEDS.

If you are like me and grieving the loss of your identity, your relationships, your job, and your sense of safety and security, I hope this book helps you find a path to regain the strength, courage, and resilience to rise up. In it I offer my best strategies for dealing with ongoing chronic illness and regaining control. My goal here is to share in a simple, accessible way the resources, tips, and tools I have learned on my journey with hEDS and some of its comorbidities. No matter where you are on your journey, there are nuggets in here that offer you wisdom, ideas to test out, or glimmers of hope for a brighter future.

The advice contained in these pages runs the gamut of physical, emotional, social, and spiritual resources that culminate in a unique recipe for a happy and healthy life – one that can help you overcome your mental and physical struggles with chronic pain and incurable illness. Knowledge and self-management skills are power. A positive approach to problem-solving and decision-making will aid in keeping your sense of independence.

In the chapters that follow you'll find an easy-to-follow healing methodology with tips for how to focus on wellness and stress reduction through rest, relaxation, and mindfulness. Like an old family recipe for a purpose-driven life, I share the right ingredients for happiness and teach you through step-by-step instructions the "secret sauce" for healing.

The culmination of habits outlined in this book changed my life. I did not plan for a life with EDS (like any of us did, right?). But these tools represent how I learned to live my best life with EDS and not be defined by it. Despite some tough long-term challenges, I continue to rise above, seek help, and get proper treatment to improve my overall quality of life. I purposefully use the behaviors and actions found in the daily habits and activities below to instill discipline in my self-care. I have achieved astonishing results, and I'm convinced they can do the same for you.

If you've picked up this book, there's one thing for certain you know: There is no silver bullet solution, no magic pill or therapy that works 100 percent of the time. That's why the patient-inspired toolkit I've created for you doesn't just have individual tools but recommendations for how to use them in concert with each other or variations of each (like a pupu platter). What I use changes day-to-day; some days I can't do physical therapy or exercise, and all I can manage is a shower and squeezing in some meditation to ease the pain. Included in these pages is advice for learning to recognize which tools are called for, which is just as important as having the tool in your toolkit.

WHY THE ZEBRA MASCOT?

By following this path I was able to discover the proverbial "pony in the pile of shit." Only it wasn't a pony – it was a Zebra – the mascot people with EDS have adopted. I continue to be extremely grateful to all my EDS friends on social media, forums, and support groups who have supported me on this book-writing journey. I involved many of you in decisions about the book, such as selecting the title and the cover design. I thank you for all your feedback and input. I wrote this for us: by a patient, for a patient. No matter where you are in your journey – new to the disease, not yet diagnosed, or maybe many years in and well versed – I hope you find something within to move you forward.

Why has the EDS community adopted the zebra mascot? In medical school, students learn the phrase "Think horses, not zebras, when you hear the sound of hooves" as part of their education to become doctors. Medical professionals use the term "zebra" to describe a very rare illness. To prevent patients from being misdiagnosed with unusual illnesses, doctors are instructed to assume that the simplest explanation is typically correct. Doctors learn to anticipate the most prevalent ailments. But as a result, many doctors appear to forget that zebras *do* exist, making it more difficult for patients with unusual diseases to receive diagnosis and treatment. EDS victims are referred to as "medical zebras" because the disorder is not easily recognizable. We all have distinct symptoms and different presentations of the condition, and even within families, it can be quite varied. Every zebra in the wild has a unique stripe pattern, much like every human has a unique set of fingerprints. The same is true for everyone suffering from EDS, and the EDS community – identifying one another by our stripes – has come together in online forums and organizations and embraced the zebra identity.

How this book is organized

This book is organized into five sections. The first is about my journey to being correctly diagnosed, the process by which people get diagnosed in general, and an overview of some common comorbidities of hypermobility. The second addresses the emotional challenge of coping with a chronic illness such as EDS, including unresolved pain and frustration and how to overcome these challenges.

The third part delves into the most critical aspect of healing – reducing stress that will finally allow the body and the mind to resume its normal healing processes. In the fourth section, I examine habits that can restore your body to better functioning with EDS including modalities of gentle exercise, nutrition, and physiotherapy. The fifth section concludes with ways you can learn to live your best life possible by prioritizing self-care, nurturing helpful relationships with others, and where to find more support in the community. At the end of the book you will also find a collection of resources, including advocacy leaders' insights, medical specialist interviews with well-known EDS experts, and information on filing for disability from a disability lawyer. I am honored to include these interviews and deeply grateful to these individuals for sharing their wisdom beyond the experiences of one patient.

Each of the chapters in parts 3–5 outline a healing habit I call my "Ms." It starts with managing pain, the medical system, and setting the proper mindset. From there, I expand on how to manage stress, autonomic dysfunction, and how to bring mindfulness and even meditation to your approach. Next, I focus on the physical body, moving away from the aspects led by your mind, to see how movement, meals, minerals, and methods such as massage and physiotherapy can help. I end by speaking to the matters of the soul where you can learn to prioritize and optimize your goals to rekindle your relationship with yourself and others.

At the end of each chapter, I prompt you to take action to help yourself because how you cope with chronic illness is within some of your control and you have a choice to make on how to proceed forward. I offer three choices – the triple A of rescue from chronic illness. They are three simple yet different ways to approach it – through your head, your heart, or your hands. With your head you can ponder to gain more self-awareness and to **assess** potential changes logically. Or through your hands you can consider taking **act**ion and move forward in your self-advocacy. And if you're not quite ready yet, try to re**affirm** to yourself that you are growing and changing for the better by repeating a strong affirmation to yourself regularly that supports your ongoing health and healing.

You may choose to skim over the medical data described in laymen's terms in the early chapters if you are well versed (or don't skip it if you're newly diagnosed). Consider jumping right into the healing habits in the latter part of the book to refresh ideas on small ways you can help yourself. Or use the index to look up specicifc topics such as comorbidities, specific tips on types of treatment, or other coping mechanisms to try.

Change is hard, and progress does not mean perfect. I have spent so much time gathering together data, research, and other insights on EDS that I am compelled to share it with you in this book. You will see imperfections, errors, and occasional typos in the book. That has been part of my process—to be all right with being imperfect. I do not expect any of us to be perfect. Progress forward is the goal. If you can take one element and start to address it, you can start to regain your sense of self and well-being for the better.

While the long journey to finally achieving a diagnosis can provide a sense of relief, it can also bring fear, frustration, anger, and despair. However, many of the symptoms once analyzed are predictable, explainable, and can be self-managed to some extent by learning what and how things affect you and how best to make effective use of treatments and advice given by your care team.

A Poem — "What If?"

Written for those of us who struggle with health issues by my friend Cliona Molloy

What if my world turns upside down
With fear and worry pulling so strong
What if I do or say something wrong
Or fail miserably letting everyone down
What if my body doesn't work so well
Impairing my independence, taking too long
What if I'm misunderstood and judged just for being me
When others don't understand difference, diversity
What if anxiety takes hold and I flee
To a place that is lonely where there is only me
What if no one will notice or understand
When I am trying my best, when I am showing my hand
Or......
What If my world was peaceful and calm
With acceptance, presence, and relative balm
Because all the *What If's* don't happen as planned!
Being in the now, reducing the load
Letting go of the past – letting the future unfold
What if I fail every so often but learn
That life is about lessons, growth, and return
To the present moment where reality sits
Accepting my body and mind
with all the quirky bits
Not seeking perfection but enjoying what's good,

Not seeking acceptance from other's but
helping them learn
What if
Difference is beautiful, diversity is key
To the freedom, wellness, and unity of all humanity,
What if
I accept and celebrate being Me

PART I

ONE PATIENT'S PERSPECTIVE

In the opening chapters I share my story of how I came to realize I had EDS. It was a 17-year-long journey filled with moments of frustration, despair, and finally hope. I share it not because my case is typical – there are no typical cases of EDS – but because in charting my journey you will understand better the conclusions I've come to and why I think the solutions I propose might help someone whose journey was different than mine. In talking with the community of zebras I've come to realize that we have so much shared wisdom among us that needs to get out and a lack of resources to aid our travels. Writing this book has been my effort to share what I know, but what I know is based on what I've experienced, and therefore it's important for you to know where I'm coming from.

I also want to make it clear that in these next three chapters I'm not engaged in some kind of "suffering Olympics" and that sharing my story is not intended to elicit pity or sympathy. I share it because parts will be familiar to some, and other aspects (like my diagnosis of craniocervical instability) are fairly rare. By showing the wide range of comorbidities I want to highlight the various ways EDS can manifest while also sharing some background about the disease in general. As a disorder of the connective tissue and because of the fact that connective tissue is found everywhere in your body, it can be hard to diagnose and treat the multisystemic nature of the symptoms hEDS causes, so my story may vary greatly from yours. But there will be elements you can relate to and resources you can utilize on your journey and for those you may care for.

CHAPTER 1

MY STORY

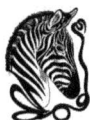

The next time you're faced with a change you didn't choose, instead of asking:
Why me? What did I do to deserve this? Why now? I am not ready for this...
Ask yourself: How is this pushing me to progress? What new experiences and opportunities will this bring? What can I do to be ready for this?

– Tuseet Jha

Everyone facing a chronic illness has a story, and too many of us understand the pain, frustration, and loneliness that come with a chronic condition. Even if we don't have a chronic condition, we can all appreciate and empathize with how it feels to struggle physically, emotionally, and financially. Maybe we gave care to someone we loved who was struggling with medical and/or other issues. No matter what our situation, we can be here for each other. Whether you are the patient, parent, child, loved one, compassionate friend, or caregiver, all of our stories are important.

This book is the story of my journey, shared with you in the hopes that you don't have to go through the same things that I did and that you find your way to the path of healing and recovery faster. I learned most of the lessons the hard way as chronic illness derailed my life and nearly cost me everything in my life that I loved.

Why EDS is such a mystery

Although I never had a name for why I was so flexible growing up nor an explanation for why my whole body seemed double-jointed, hypermobility had been present my whole life. I just thought I was good at yoga! As a young athlete, I was prone to injury and had a lot of growing pains; after becoming an adult, I had a strange array of health issues, but no one could ever put a name to what I was experiencing. Because doctors couldn't figure me out, I was frequently dismissed as crazy; often they chalked up my symptoms as related to "women's issues," first saying it was due to my weight and then that I was depressed. I have literally gone to the ER in pain from hypermobility only to be sent home and told to "drink a glass of wine and get over it."

Many years ago things got so bad that my doctors sent me to be evaluated at the National Institutes of Health. Specialists ran multiple tests and ultimately diagnosed me with Hashimoto's autoimmune thyroid issues. The only evidence they could find of something wrong with me was that the antibodies in my blood were off the charts – that I had an autoimmune issue. No one back then was studying connective tissue disorders like hypermobility (arguably not much now either, but that is changing). Doctors warned me I might develop multiple sclerosis, lupus, or even things I had never heard of before like Sjögren's syndrome.

AUTOIMMUNE DISEASE

Many chronic illnesses are autoimmune disorders, such as MS, lupus, and type 1 diabetes. These are conditions in which the immune system attacks the body itself, and according to Harvard medical, they **affect one of every 15 Americans.** While autoimmune diseases can appear quite different in each individual, they share fundamental characteristics. Autoimmunity means that cells within your body are attacking your own healthy cells, often causing irreparable damage. But such issues can be hard to identify and even harder to address (how can you fight a disease when you're already fighting yourself?). Worse yet is the fact that when you get one autoimmune disease, you're highly likely to develop others as well, as your cells target other organs or systems, leading to new and different diagnoses. Managing an autoimmune disease can be a lifelong journey.

With each new diagnosis, I assumed I had the answer. But life went on, and my quality of life deteriorated. I thought I was just tired when I started regularly running off the road, assuming I was dozing off on my hour-long commute. I didn't think much of it at the time as a good night's sleep was just one of many things that had disappeared over these years; that is until one day when the realization that something was seriously wrong with me when the wheel of my steering wheel of my car literally hit me in the face. I had fallen asleep on the highway and had crashed into a back of a car that was stopped dead in traffic. That was the end of my life as I knew it.

The severe neck injuries I sustained ultimately revealed that I was losing consciousness while driving not because of fatigue but due to a lack of blood flow to my brain. It wasn't just that my joints were flexible: The stretchy nature of my veins meant that they expanded instead of carrying my blood upwards against the pull of gravity to my brain. I had become a living Mrs. Incredible – ElastiGirl – but my superpower meant that instead of proper circulation my blood pooled in my feet and my ankles turned purple. Combined with the fact that I could now sublux or dislocate multiple joints in my spine with simple movements finally led to a life-altering discovery. Hiding underneath and connecting all my underlying medical issues was a newfound diagnosis: I had hypermobile Ehlers-Danlos syndrome (hEDS).

Why EDS is so debilitating

I knew a little about EDS already because a few of my family members had it. It turns out this is not surprising, as EDS is genetically passed down through the generations. However, unlike the family silver, this inheritance was a mystery. It had a name, but little else was understood about the condition, much less how to live with and learn how to manage it.

I came to learn that EDS is a very complex multisystemic genetic disorder linked to faulty collagen – the main protein found in skin, tendons, ligaments, cartilage, connective tissue, and even bone. Collagen is found basically everywhere in your body and is essentially responsible for "holding" you together. People suffering from EDS quite literally start falling apart.

In my case, not content to just shut off the flow of blood to my brain, EDS also began messing with my heart. I was soon diagnosed with another blood circulation condition – postural orthostatic tachycardia syndrome (POTS) – causing my heart rate to spike upon standing or moving to an upright position. POTS is a disorder of the autonomic nervous system, essentially triggering a constant "fight-or-flight" response. My whole body was in hyper-adrenal chronic overdrive – a panic attack on steroids that was 24/7.

If that wasn't enough, one day my neurologist realized that my head was falling off – no kidding. EDS and the car wreck had so weakened my neck that my skull was beginning to slide off the top of my spinal cord, causing craniocervical instability and the beginnings of mild Chiari. In laymen's terms, the prolonged stress and strain of the simple act of holding my head up was causing my brain to drop down onto my brain stem at the base of my skull, wreaking havoc with my spinal cord and causing irreversible brain damage.

I tried to hide the severity of what I was feeling from my husband and my daughter, but soon I was barely able to function. It got to the point where I could not walk straight, climb the stairs, or even finish a sentence. Unable to work anymore, I had to go on disability. As a career-focused woman, I was devastated when several members of my care team told me that I would likely never work again. But it wasn't until I developed a heart embolism that I finally got the message – that and my doctor pulling me aside and bluntly saying, "You have to change your life or you will die before your next birthday."

And so began the research project of my life – to find a path forward for myself and others afflicted with hEDS.

Why EDS is hard to treat

It didn't take long to realize that there was a lack of resources available for chronic illnesses and invisible diseases such as EDS. I searched high and low for answers, seeking out expert doctors, advanced care specialists, and leading-edge medical research hospitals to get on year-long waiting lists to be seen by them, only to be dismissed by most and repeatedly told "EDS is too complex to treat."

Many of us spend years searching for answers or for a diagnosis that fits. Everywhere I looked turned out to be a dead end. By comparison, the decision to undergo multi-level spinal fusion and brain decompression surgery to "put my head on straight" was a no-brainer. I was petrified to be sure, but at least the doctors had answers. No one that I could discover had an answer to EDS. If I wanted one I was going to have to find it out for myself.

It's hard to believe, but there is no single treatment and there are no EDS specialist doctors (yet). It takes a village. However, the answers I have found came from trial and error, thousands of hours of research with input from many patients in the zebra community who also are desperately seeking solutions.

And so I began to study my condition and learn everything I could about it. I took courses on any topic (such as movement classes in tai chi and qigong) that I thought might help contribute to my recovery and looked into subjects as diverse as aqua therapy and mindfulness – anything I thought might help me regain capabilities and achieve not just a tolerable but a good quality of life. I took my time exploring these topics and wound up completely overhauling my lifestyle and changing my ideas about rest, nutrition, and exercise.

Over time EDS manifested itself in a multitide of different ways. I started the process of documenting the changes and their impact on my symptoms while analyzing the long-term effect of my attempts to respond and counter its effects. I looked at EDS comprehensively, examining the full scope of wellness approaches – naturally, medically, pharmaceutically, mentally, physically, and emotionally. The chapters that follow outline my path. Along the way I discovered several modalities that worked, and I stuck with them daily, watching my weakened body slowly but surely grow stronger every day.

Several years later my cardiologist sat in amazement as he listened to my heart calmly beat out its rhythm, down to only 50 beats per minute from the previous 150 bpm average. How could I have possibly beaten a lifelong and oftentimes debilitating condition like POTS and repaired the damage my heart suffered from the embolism I had? "You are a living miracle," he said. But it wasn't a miracle: It was combining multiple methods to calm my body down and decompress the tension I had been carrying all those years.

Why I wrote this book

My story might have ended there. I was on a path to recovery and knew that if I remained committed, I would continue to heal and find ways to flourish despite EDS. But my real breakthrough came when I realized that through learning how to heal myself, I could help others by sharing my experience, the lessons I learned, and the resources I discovered – turning my health journey into mind and body wellness for others with EDS. I found I was happier and profoundly less stressed when I focused on the big picture instead of just my problems. I had not had this level of energy or drive to *really* build something in any of my previous jobs or former roles. This offered me a truly higher purpose: my pain could be transformed into something that helped others. I had something to gain from my losses; they had given me strength, the courage to heal, and a passion for helping others.

Certainly some of my enthusiasm stemmed from the positive feedback I was receiving about the changes others were seeing in me. People wanted to know what I had done. I was given the opportunity to share my experience from a patient's perspective on "How I Saved My Own Life" at the 2021 EDS educational annual conference. Many doctors also recognized my successes, and my cardiologist encouraged me to offer workshops to his patients and their families to see if they too could achieve similar goals. As part of my outreach, I even created a small business called Journey2Joy and started offering free classes online that focused on helping chronically ill and disabled people. I helped a few grateful people, and some even became good friends.

But my new purpose allowed me to let go of the approval-seeking and people-pleasing outlook of looking externally to meet my needs for feeling loved and worthy. Now I live life with a sense I am serving more than my limited self in sharing what I've learned with others. I discovered in making different choices and changing old habits that I was driven by courage and that with perseverance and resilience I could retrain my brain from negative thinking to a positive growth mindset. As my journey continues, I am awake to a higher purpose that permits a more authentic me to emerge, utilizing my inner strengths to seek the joy in living.

I offer you this book in the hopes of giving you the wisdom, insight, tools, and tips to learn to cope and even thrive with chronic illness. The EDS community is full of wonderful people who compassionately share their struggles, and that compassion was crucial to my healing and hopefully will be to yours. If this book helps even one person more quickly arrive at the right diagnosis, set out on their journey of recovery, achieve a sense of balance and wellness, or leave feeling a little less alone, it will have been worth it.

Choose to Assess, Act, or Affirm

- **Assess:** Is it hard to think that an optimistic attitude might be a factor in helping yourself in some way? Try not to feel dismissed, but allow the spark of imagination to inspire hopefulness in your soul.

- **Act:** Can you permit yourself to think of one good thing that has come into your life due to your illness or your diagnosis?

- **Affirm**: "I love the parts of me that need love the most right now. By unearthing the core reason I am suffering, I illuminate the path to sustained well-being."

NOTES

CHAPTER 2

EDS AND ME

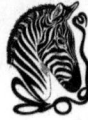

When life doesn't go to plan, we must embrace the change and realize that our lives are composed of chapters; one has ended, and another one is about to begin. But we can't move on to the next chapter if we continually re-read old ones. We have to willingly accept that life goes on and that we have a chance to create something bigger and better.

– Adam Bergen

If you are just starting out learning more about EDS or were recently diagnosed, this is all new to you and can be quite overwhelming. The Internet can be a good place to start to learn about hypermobility, but it is important to consider that not all information is of equal standard. Let's start with the basics from credible sources. The syndrome derives its name from clinical case reports presented by two physicians who were dermatologists: in 1901 Edvard Ehlers recognized the condition as a distinct entity, and later in 1908 Henri-Alexandre Danlos suggested that skin extensibility and fragility were the cardinal features of the syndrome. The international nonprofit Ehlers-Danlos Society describes EDS as follows:

> The Ehlers-Danlos syndromes (EDS) are a group of hereditary disorders of connective tissue that are varied in the ways they affect the body and in their genetic causes. The underlying concern is the abnormal structure or function of collagen and certain allied connective tissue proteins. They are generally characterized by joint hyper-mobility (joints that move further than normal range), joint instability (subluxation defined as a partial separation of the articulating sur-faces of a joint) and dislocations (full separation of the surfaces of a joint), scoliosis, and other joint deformities, skin hyperextensibility (skin that can be stretched further than normal) and abnormal scarring, and other structural weak-ness such as hernias and organ prolapse through the pelvic floor.

EDS in short affects the body's connective tissue. Connective tissue lies between other tissues and organs, keeping these separate while connecting and supporting them, holding everything in place, including skin, tendons, ligaments, blood vessels, internal organs, and bones. Connective tissue is vital in every system and every organ, greatly affecting every aspect of life. You can now realize why your entire body is affected by this disease!

The different types of EDS

There are 13 subtypes of EDS, the most recent discovered in 2018. Hypermobile EDS (hEDS) is the most common type. Other types of EDS include classical EDS, vascular EDS, and kyphoscoliotic EDS. Different tissues and organs can be affected in diverse ways depending on the genetic fault in the collagen and proteins, which explains why there are several subtypes of EDS. At its root, however, EDS is caused by a genetic mutation in a certain kind of connective tissue – the variety will depend on the type of EDS but usually a form of collagen – causing it to be fragile and stretchy. This stretchiness can sometimes be seen in the skin of someone with EDS (i.e., wrinkles or cellulite) but not always. Many individuals with the condition are hypermobile – able to extend one or more of their joints further than is usual. This is why we are known as being flexible, bendy, or double-jointed. As collagen is present throughout the body, people with EDS tend to experience a broad range of symptoms that are less visible than the skin and joint differences. This often causes symptoms in organ systems where hyperextension can cause injury, long-term pain, aching muscles, and chronic fatigue. Blood circulation is reduced causing dizziness, palpitations, and digestive disorders. Other symptoms can result in blood pressure issues and loss of mobility to even hair changes or dental issues. These are complex syndromes affecting many systems of the body at once. Despite this, EDS is often an invisible disability as many patients look "normal." Such problems and their severity vary considerably from person to person and even in the same type of EDS and within the same family. (Learn more about the diagnostic criteria for the 13 subtypes of EDS at https://www.ehlers-danlos.com/eds-types/; The EDS Support UK website has more information about the different types of EDS at https://www.ehlers-danlos.org/what-is-eds/information-on-eds/types-of-eds/.)

Because the disorder can affect different body systems, its wide-ranging symptoms can remain unconnected for many years. There can be a wide range of severity of symptoms and concerns within each type of EDS, and each person's case of Ehlers-Danlos syndrome will be unique. There are also overlapping symptoms that can sometimes look like Lyme disease, chronic fatigue, or fibromyalgia. That may lead to misdiagnosis or delayed treatment and ineffective or inappropriate therapies. As a result, **on average it takes *a dozen years* for patients with EDS to get a proper diagnosis.** The gene mutations causing all of the subtypes have been identified and can be tested for except hypermobile EDS.

Although there is no cure for the Ehlers-Danlos syndromes, once diagnosed there is treatment for symptoms, and there are preventative measures that are helpful for most if you can find the proper care and you look at your body's health issues holistically. Learning self-management skills can help you and your health care team build a partnership to support you when you need it as your condition changes or flares up. The prognosis depends on the type of Ehlers-Danlos syndrome and the individual. People with Ehlers-Danlos syndrome (EDSers) may have a higher risk for infections due to their fragile skin's inability to quickly heal. EDSers often have a lowered immune system function, possibly due to chronic stress on multiple body systems or an lgG3 deficiency.

EDS can affect people in different ways. For some, the condition is relatively mild, while for others their symptoms worsen over time, with joint pain and instability leading to reduced function and quality of life. This might occur because they have not received the right advice, treatments have not been effective, or treatments have only been able to slow down a natural tendency in that person for their condition to worsen. For other people, treatment or surgeries can significantly improve their well-being, function, and quality of life, or hold them in a steady state so that they no longer feel they are deteriorating and are able to better manage their concerns. Some of the rare and severe types can be life-threatening, but for most EDSers life expectancy is normal, although day-to-day living can be challenging. Whereas some of the risks and consequences cannot be controlled, it is helpful to recognize that many aspects can be self-managed with lifestyle planning, changes, and appropriate health care support.

Who gets EDS

Current research says the overall prevalence of EDS is between 1 in 3,500 to 1 in 5,000 people. Dr. Chip Norris at the Medical University at South Carolina (MUSC) and his team theorize that it is more like 1 in 500 based on his patient registry of DNA samples and genetic research.

The main way EDS is inherited is autosomal dominant inheritance – it's genetically passed on to you, which is why I call it genetic trauma. While Some people? carry EDS in their DNA, for many, the onset of problematic symptoms and a diagnosis don't come until later after a bodily trauma, such as a car accident, or catching a severe flu, virus, or other event triggers it. Until then, many experience hypermobility and other symptoms that are not properly associated with EDS. (It's my working theory that a post-viral load or a triggering event can kick it off.)

For others, hypermobility issues appear to emerge with puberty, while female athletes seem to be able to postpone the onset of EDS because they maintain excellent muscle tone to compensate for the faulty collagen and ligaments. Women, especially young teens, are more prone to early development of the illness. Several sex hormones begin to increase in production during puberty, affecting the entire body. Boys and girls have distinct hormone levels and they can also vary from person to person and throughout time. Of the 70 percent of women who had hEDS symptoms before puberty, a little over half said puberty made them worse. This could be because human organs and other components have estradiol (estrogen) receptors, including joints, skin, and cartilage. For example, anterior cruciate ligament (ACL) laxity rises with increased estrogen and progesterone levels during a woman's regular menstrual cycle. ACL ruptures in female athletes are 2–8 times more common than in male athletes. At the same time, many older women get sick later in life, often postpartum or after menopause. There is a possible hormonal link to its start, although no medical research has confirmed it.

The faulty gene that causes EDS is passed on by one parent, and there's a 50 percent risk of each child to develop the condition. Sometimes the faulty gene is not inherited but occurs in the person for the first time. Its genetic cause means that a child cannot inherit a different kind of EDS from the one their parent has; it also means that one type cannot later turn into another, and there is no increased risk of having another type just because you have one. The severity of the condition can vary within the same family.

Knowing that your child may have EDS may come as a shock, a relief that your child's seemingly unconnected problems had a name, or simply a confirmation of what you previously thought. It will take time for you to acclimatize to the news and then face daily life with EDS in the best way for you and your child. One of the most important things you can do to aid your child is to educate yourself on EDS, its types, and severity. This will help you decide how to best support your child's needs.

Current knowledge of hypermobile EDS

The most common type of EDS is thought to be the hypermobile type (formerly known as the hypermobility type, or type 3). As Dr. Norris explains, "Generalized joint hypermobility, impacting four or more joints, has been reported to be present in anywhere from 12 to 28 percent of children, adolescents, and young adults. This has been shown to be both age and gender-specific, where females and children tend to be more hypermobile." As the name suggests, hypermobility is the ability to have your joints move beyond their typical range, causing pain as well as joint instability and often very tight or strained muscles.

New criteria for diagnosing hypermobile EDS (hEDS) were published in the 2017 EDS International Classification. According to the EDS Society, to be diagnosed with hEDS, one needs to meet three separate groups of criteria below:

1. An assessment of present and historical hypermo-bility using a scoring system called the Beighton score. At present it is the only standard used commonly to test hypermobile joints. The Beighton score is a simple 9-point system to quantify joint laxity and range of motion, where the higher the score, the higher the laxity, with the threshold varying for younger versus older individuals.

2. The second criterion is divided into three features. To meet this criterion, an individual must meet two of these three features.

a. Having at least five from a list of 12 signs and symptoms that can be identified by physical examination and additional testing. These signs and symptoms include soft/velvety/stretchy skin, stretchmarks, hernias, prolapse of organs (when they slip down from their normal position), and/or mitral valve prolapse.

b. Having a close family member (parent, child, brother, or sister) who independently meets the criteria for a diagnosis of hypermobile EDS, though they may have different and variable symptoms.

c. Having significant pain or unstable joints recurring daily for at least 3 months.

3. Other types of EDS and related connective tissue disorders need to have been considered by a doctor and ruled out.

The 2017 EDS International Classification defined for the first time some related conditions known as hypermobility spectrum disorders (HSD), which have similar symptoms to hEDS (the term "joint hypermobility syndrome" ([JHS]) is no longer used). The US medical diagnosis code for hypermobile Ehlers-Danlos syndrome is ICD-10-CM Diagnosis Code Q79.62 (more information can be found at https://www.icd10data.com/ICD10CM/Codes/Q00-Q99/Q65-Q79/Q79-/Q79.62).

For more insights on identifying hypermobile EDS, the Ehlers-Danlos Society has a quick and easy checklist for evaluating if you might have hEDS at https://www.ehlers-danlos.com/wp-content/uploads/hEDS-Dx-Criteria-checklist-1-Fillable-form.pdf. Although the 2017 classification is a big improvement, one of the most helpful resources on hEDS is the 2020 book *Disjointed: Navigating the Diagnosis and Management of hypermobile Ehlers-Danlos Syndrome and Hypermobility Spectrum Disorders,* which has contributions from several EDS-knowledgeable experts and specialized doctors. It is an incredible (almost encyclopedic) resource for EDS patients. I strongly recommend the book when you want to learn deep knowledge from the medical community and research perspective. (One caveat – many say it's the best book out there on EDS, but it's so heavy we can hardly hold it in our hypermobile hands!) Claire Smith's book, *Understanding Hypermobile Ehlers-Danlos Syndrome and Hypermobility Spectrum Disorder*, written in 2017, is very helpful in understanding hypermobility, its origins, and where it stood in the medical landscape at the time she wrote the book. Her book is a very insightful resource on the diagnosis and many of its comorbidities.

Common symptoms of hEDS

Many things about the multi- and cross-systematic symptoms of hEDS make it very difficult to diagnose. It can present very differently from person to person, change over time, and vary in severity. There are many symptoms common to hEDS, including those on the list below:

- Joint instability, hyper-extensions, subluxations, and dislocations;
- History of musculoskeletal problems and injuries;
- Chronic pain;
- Chronic fatigue;
- Cardiovascular problems;
- Skin that is stretchier or softer than normal;
- Obstetrics and gynecological issues with the pelvic floor;
- Easily bruised;
- Poor wound healing;
- Flat feet or fallen arches;
- Bladder issues;
- Abnormal scarring;
- Poor proprioception;
- Dental issues;
- Allergies and/or mast cell abnormalities;
- Autoimmunity;
- Scoliosis;
- Varicose veins.

I experience many areas of joint instability and frequent subluxations, causing chronic pain in the neck at all my cervical joints, both right and left hip sockets, sacroiliac (SI) joints, and in my spine. Regular head movements can cause easy joint subluxation, causing muscle spasms and pain. I require several hours of bracing daily for my neck and hips, often sleeping in soft braces. My ribs frequently come out as well and can take days to go back in. Even my wrist pops out of the socket leading to tendonitis and requiring a soft brace, which makes it very hard to type these words!

I am easily bruised and struggle with wounds and scarring that will not heal properly. I also have common EDS skin issues – not with elasticity that is so often pictured but strange marks, bumps, and unknown redness sometimes seen. And I have multiple joint disc degeneration and herniation in the neck and at numerous locations along my entire spine, leading to the diagnosis of scoliosis in my back.

The symptoms of hEDS are very complex and can be very challenging to treat. Often patients are riddled with multiple comorbidities of other aligning diagnoses, including heart and autonomic dysfunction, rheumatological impairments such as lupus, and autoimmune disease. Researchers are even looking into a possible relationship between autism and EDS. Unfortunately, there is a lot of overlap in these different conditions and their symptoms, making diagnosis even harder. Here are some of the more common issues experienced by those with hEDS:

- The autonomic nervous system can cause a wide variability in the heart rate and blood pressure, contributing to a hyper-state of an overactive sympathetic nervous system. This disruption can cause symptoms and complaints in patients, including sleep trouble, digestive issues, energy and fatigue, and cognitive issues.

- The gastrointestinal system can create problems with food processing (called motility), food sensitivities, and other bowel conditions.

- The immune system causes hyper-reactive responses to foods, chemicals, temperatures, or other triggers.

- The peripheral nervous system causes numbness, pain, and tingling in the extremities.

Unfortunately, because hEDS affects the connective tissue that supports muscles, tendons, cartilage, and bones, sufferers can often stretch their joints and skin beyond normal limits during pregnancy, potentially affecting the mother and fetus. The increased flexibility of tissues can offer extra challenges for hypermobile women that require careful planning and control.

Symptoms worsened for 26 percent of women during pregnancy and 37 percent afterward. Premature birth, placenta previa, and cervical insufficiency are all risks for pregnant women with EDS. Many persons with hEDS report that their pain symptoms began during their first pregnancy, and pregnancy-induced laxity may not settle properly postnatally.

In my case, I was bedridden during most of my only pregnancy and had to deliver early due to blood pressure abnormalities and preeclampsia. My body's method of signaling something was wrong was to faint and throw up, so I was induced and faced emergency labor. Many of my early symptoms of hEDS started during pregnancy and increased postpartum. But at the time I ascribed it to the stress my body was under and the major lifestyle changes a newborn brings. It's only now that I realize dysautonomia – one of the major comorbidities of hEDS (see below) was at work even then.

Researchers advise doctors to take preventative steps to avoid premature births and to order further tests to assure the mother's and the baby's safety. Your general practitioner, midwife, and other health professionals should be kept informed of your progress as well as your lifestyle changes, and you should give your caregivers a birth plan that includes unique considerations and precautions for your joints and skin. With the aid of your health care team, you may make it a joyful experience with minimal complications.

In some countries, other specialists or even GPs may be able to order blood tests, urine tests, or skin biopsies to confirm certain types of EDS. In the case of hEDS, any doctor can make a clinical diagnosis by going through the diagnostic checklist. Referrals to a rheumatologist or geneticist might be necessary if an acquired connective tissue disease (e.g., lupus) or a rarer type of EDS needs to be excluded. There are still no reliable genetic tests to conclusively diagnose hEDS, although Dr. Chip Norris and his team at the Norris Lab (www.thenorrislab.com)

at MUSC are working diligently to change that. They are on the cutting edge of this work and hope to soon publish in a peer-reviewed medical journal their discovery of the genetic marker(s) of hypermobile EDS. You can read more about what researchers and scientists are doing at MUSC to develop a blood test in my interview in the Appendix with Dr. Norris and his primary research student, Cortney Gensemer, who has EDS herself.

An EDS diagnosis can put all the pieces of the puzzle together and connect the dots. As Dr. Heidi Collins said many years ago at an EDS conference to help doctors recognize the various symptoms, "If you can't connect the issues, think connective tissues." Knowing for certain if you have EDS gives you and your medical team some idea of where problems can come from and why they are happening. As more people are diagnosed, EDS and HSD are gaining the attention needed to increase care, education, and research, hopefully leading to better health outcomes.

Choose to Assess, Act, or Affirm

- **Assess:** What potentially new symptoms did you notice in this chapter that you have been experiencing and maybe not yet realized? Take note and discuss with your doctors.

- **Act:** What follow-up medical appointments should you schedule to further your understanding and evaluation?

- **Affirm:** "My peace is more powerful than my pain."

Bibliography

Casanova, E. L., Baeza-Velasco, C., Buchanan, C. B., and Casanova, M. F. (2020). "The Relationship between Autism and Ehlers-Danlos Syndromes/Hypermobility Spectrum Disorders." *Journal of Personalized Medicine*, 10(4), 260. https://doi.org/10.3390/jpm10040260.

Heitz, N. A., Eisenman, P. A., Beck, C. L., and Walker, J. A. (1999). "Hormonal Changes throughout the Menstrual Cycle and Increased Anterior Cruciate Ligament Laxity in Females." *Journal of Athletic Training*, 34(2), 144–149.

Hugon-Rodin, J., et al. (2016). "Gynecologic Symptoms and the Influence on Reproductive Life in 386 Women with Hypermobility type Ehlers-Danlos Syndrome: A Cohort Study." *Orphanet J Rare Dis* 11(124). https://doi.org/10.1186/s13023-016-0511-2.

Jovin, Diana (Ed.). (2020). *Disjointed: Navigating the Diagnosis and Management of Hypermobile Ehlers-Danlos Syndrome and Hypermobility Spectrum Disorders*. Hidden Stripes Publishing.

Smith, Claire. (2017). *Understanding Hypermobile Ehlers-Danlos Syndrome and Hypermobility Spectrum Disorder*. Redcliff House Publications.

"What are the Ehlers-Danlos Syndromes?" (n.d.). *The Ehlers Danlos Society*. https://www.ehlers-danlos.com/what-is-eds/.

NOTES

CHAPTER 3

COMORBIDITIES OF EDS

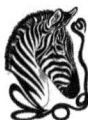

---

*Sometimes, all you can do is accept there's not much
you can do. And sometimes all you can control is
how well you let go of control.*

— **Lori Deschene**

If EDS wasn't enough, oftentimes those with hEDS experience what's come to be known as the "trifecta" — the all-too-common comorbidities of dysautonomia/ POTS and mastocytosis/mast cell activation syndrome (MCAS). Other than the fact that these disorders are prevalent comorbidities, research has not yet shown any link between joint hypermobility and their occurrence. I talk about both below, though my discussion of the latter is more limited because I do not suffer from mast cell activation. However, I have experienced craniocervical instability, which I discuss in more detail here as well.

Dysautonomia, POTS, and orthostatic intolerance

The nonprofit Dysautonomia International describes postural orthostatic tachycardia syndrome (POTS) as a form of dysautonomia that is estimated to affect between one and three million Americans and millions more around the world. (You can learn more about this organization in my interview with their co-founder and president, Lauren Stiles, in the Appendix.) POTS causes dizziness due to an unusually high increase in heart rate when standing (a healthy individual has a slight increase in heart rate – about 10–15 beats per minute (bpm) – within the first 10 minutes of standing). Orthostatic intolerance is a general term for several conditions in which symptoms are made worse by upright posture and improve with recumbency or laying down flat. It can be a debilitating condition that affects routine activities, such as working or attending school. POTS primarily affects women of child-bearing age, with most studies reporting a greater than 80–90 percent female predominance. The peak time line for onset is at age 14, but half of all individuals with POTS develop it in adulthood. Dysautonomia can occur as a primary condition or associated with other conditions, including EDS, Parkinson's disease, Sjögren's syndrome, or diabetes.

One way to understand this rare and unusual disease is to think of gravity's effects as blood flows through the body. When a healthy person stands, any lightheaded feeling is infrequent because the leg muscles help pump blood back up to the heart, and because the body turns on a series of reflexes. The body then releases norepinephrine and epinephrine (also known as adrenaline) to make up for the lower amount of blood returning to the heart immediately after standing. Adrenaline makes the heartbeat a little faster with more force (like when we exercise or are frightened), and norepinephrine causes the blood vessels to tighten or constrict. The result is increased blood returning to the heart and brain. The average person is completely unaware of these reflex changes in blood flow when standing.

But with someone with HEDS and POTS, blood does not correctly get constricted in loose and lax veins, limiting its ability to return to the heart as it tries to go against the pull of gravity when standing. When people with POTS stand or sit upright, they appear to pool a larger amount of blood in vessels below the heart. Compared to healthy individuals, for the person with POTS, the more time they remain upright, the more significant the proportion of their blood that settles in their abdomen and limbs. The body responds by releasing more norepinephrine or epinephrine in an attempt to cause more constriction of the blood vessels. For various reasons (not all of which are well understood), the blood vessels in people with POTS do not seem to respond normally, and the vessels either do not constrict properly or dilate. But because the heart remains able to respond to the norepinephrine and epinephrine, the heart rate increases. As a result, standing or sitting upright for those with POTS turns our extremities purple while decreasing our oxygen intake, which causes an increase in both heart rate and breathlessness, leading to dizziness, nausea, and even syncope (passing out temporarily due to a lack of blood flow to the brain). The result can be a feeling of unease, lightheadedness, seeing stars, darkening of vision, or even fainting – like when I passed out while driving.

Many doctors used to believe POTS was caused by anxiety, but research has since ruled that out. It turns out that POTS has many causes with similar clinical manifestations and is not a disease; it is simply a cluster of symptoms frequently seen together. This is why the "S" in POTS stands for "syndrome." However, figuring out what is causing the symptoms of POTS in each patient can be very difficult. In many cases, patients and their doctors will not be able to determine the precise underlying cause.

One reason for the difficulty establishing an underlying cause is because symptoms vary from person to person and often are similar to those in other conditions. There is evidence that POTS can arise from abnormalities in autonomic nervous system function, immune system function including autoimmunity, blood volume and blood flow regulation, or a combination of these factors. Genetic factors probably also affect susceptibility to POTS. Many people with POTS report a preceding medical or life-changing event, such as viral infection, concussion, surgery, pregnancy, or puberty.

Common symptoms of POTS

According to my cardiologist and POTS specialist Dr. Hasan Abdallah, many common symptoms of dysautonomia can include:

- Extreme fatigue;
- Facial flushing/rosacea/acne;
- Positive allergy tests to many environmental factors (i.e., molds, trees, foods);
- Increased heart rate when standing, including feeling lightheaded and off-balance;
- Headaches/nausea;
- Constipation/bladder issues;
- Night sweats/sleep apnea;
- Anxiety/depression;
- Other Symptoms: swollen lymph node, easy bruising, trouble concentrating, high cholesterol.

Frustratingly, many of these symptoms are not correlated and lead to no particular diagnosis or are often misdiagnosed as chronic fatigue, fibromyalgia, anxiety, and/or depression. I struggled with symptoms like tachycardia, tremors, anxiety, blood pooling in my extremities, swollen ankles, and brain fog. POTS symptoms are usually triggered during:

- Prolonged upright posture (such as standing in line, standing in a shower, or even sitting at a desk for long periods);

- Being in a warm environment (such as in hot summer weather, a hot, crowded room, a hot shower or bath);
- Immediately after exercise;
- After emotionally stressful events (seeing gory scenes, being scared);
- After eating (when blood flow shifts to the intestines during digestion);
- And when fluid and salt intake are inadequate.

Some POTS patients have relatively mild symptoms and can continue routine work, school, social, and recreational activities. For others, it can be a disabling condition whose symptoms may be so severe that normal life activities, such as bathing, housework, eating, sitting upright, walking, or standing, can be significantly limited. Approximately 25 percent of POTS patients are disabled and unable to work according to Dysautonomia International. Doctors and specialty physicians, usually POTS cardiologists, have compared the functional impairment seen in POTS patients to the impairment seen in chronic obstructive pulmonary disease (COPD) or congestive heart failure. I was also diagnosed with a heart embolism during this difficult time. Researchers found that the quality of life in POTS patients is comparable to patients on dialysis for kidney failure.

Diagnosing, testing, and treatment for POTS

A challenge in obtaining a diagnosis is the shortage of POTS specialists, and those available often have long waiting lists, ranging from six months to over two years (I had to wait a year to see mine). One patient survey found that more than half of POTS patients traveled more than 100 miles from home, and over 20 percent of patients traveled more than 500 miles from home for POTS-related medical care. In the same survey, patients reported seeing an average of seven physicians before receiving a POTS diagnosis and an average diagnostic delay of almost five years.

A cardiologist familiar with POTS can diagnose it using different tests and diagnostic criteria developed by several leading medical organizations. These criteria include:

- Heart rate increases of 30 beats per minute (bpm) or more, or over 120 bpm, within the first 10 minutes of standing, in the absence of orthostatic hypotension (upon diagnosis my resting heart rate was averaging 150 bpm lying down).
- A revised standard of a 40 bpm or more increase has recently been adopted in children and adolescents.

POTS is often diagnosed by a tilt table test. During this test, you are secured on a table while lying flat. Then the table is raised to an almost upright position. Your heart rate, blood pressure, blood oxygen, and exhaled carbon dioxide levels are measured for changes. Variables of symptoms are also monitored including lightheadedness, nausea, dizziness, and pooling of blood in the extremities. For some patients, it can be intimidating and even scary

and provoke a fainting spell. However, under close monitoring and through straps keeping your body in place, this
is a routine procedure usually conducted by a trained cardiologist that is safe.

If such testing is not available, it can be analyzed with
bedside measurements of heart rate and blood pressure
taken in the supine (laying down) and standing up position
at two, five, and ten-minute intervals. Doctors may perform more detailed tests to evaluate the autonomic nervous
system in POTS patients, such as quantitative sudomotor
axon reflex test (QSART, sometimes called Q-Sweat), ther-
moregulatory sweat test (TST), skin biopsies (looking at
the small fiber nerves), gastric motility studies, and more.

**If you suspect you might have POTS, one easy at-
home evaluation is to hold one hand up at a 90-degree
angle and the other hand downward at a 90-degree
angle for 60 seconds. Then bring them back to your
middle. Does one hand look different (more swollen or
discolored) than the other? Seek medical advice if so.**

POTS is a serious condition that can significantly affect
the quality of life, but it's not usually life-threatening.
There is no permanent cure or standardized treatment protocol available for POTS, but various treatment options
are available to manage the disease.

Many people learn how to control their symptoms and
live complete and active lives. As everyone has different
symptoms and comorbidities, there is no standardized
therapy for POTS, and current treatment options focus on
addressing the symptoms that bother you most. However,

this could all be changing, mainly due to researchers Dr. William Gunning and Dr. Blair Grubb from the University of Toledo. Dr. Grubb, who has been treating POTS patients and studying the condition for more than three decades, says he believes he and his collaborators are increasingly close to proving a long-held theory that POTS is an autoimmune disorder. This could be a game changer and lead to future testing, treatments, and hope.

Mast cells, mastocytosis, and MCAS

Mast cells are the body's immune system cells that live in the bone marrow and body tissues, both internally and externally. Everyone has mast cells in their body, and they play many complex and critical roles in keeping us healthy. People have the highest numbers of mast cells where the body meets the environment: the skin, lungs, and intestinal tract. As a result, disorders with mast cells can affect the gastrointestinal system, the airway lining, and the skin.

When mast cells detect a germ or virus, they set off an inflammatory (allergic) response by releasing a chemical called histamine. This response protects your body from germs and infections. They are also involved in allergic reactions, from the tiny swelling that appears after a mosquito bite to a life-threatening, full-blown anaphylaxis where you can't breathe.

Mastocytosis is caused by an excess of mast cells gathering in the tissues of the body. It is not contagious or inherited. Unfortunately, people with mastocytosis face a high risk of developing severe reactions. Symptoms can include unexplained flushing, abdominal pain, bloating, and severe reactions to foods, medicines, dyes, or insect stings. The danger is these can seem similar to a normal allergic reaction and sometimes go undiagnosed. Mastocytosis is also rare; according to the Cleveland Clinic, it occurs in one in every 20,000 people.

MCAS (mast cell activation syndrome) is a condition in which the mast cells in the body release an inappropriate amount of chemicals into the body. Symptoms of MCAS include extreme itching, flushing, hives, reddish complexion, burning feeling, lightheadedness, dizziness, syncope, arrhythmia, tachycardia, diarrhea, nausea, vomiting, cramping, intestinal discomfort, constipation, swallowing difficulties, throat tightness, congestion, coughing, wheezing, and even anaphylaxis. MCAS is usually diagnosed through serum tests for the level of mast cell tryptase (which is a chemical they release) and/or a skin biopsy. Many symptoms of both diseases can be treated with (potentially dramatic) dietary changes and heavy doses of antihistamines, stabilizers, and corticosteroids.

For more information on mastocytosis, MCAS, and the correlations of all three conditions, check out the book *The Trifecta Passport* by Amber Walker.

Craniocervical instability

Many neurological and spinal disorders have been discovered to be more common in the brains and backs of EDS patients. It is not unusual for hypermobile EDSers to have joint instability, including in the cervical spine (i.e., the neck). When your joints, tendons, and muscular structure in your spine are not adequately supporting your bowling ball-sized head, it protrudes forward, increasing weight on the spine, which can lead to many neurological symptoms. Craniocervical instability (CCI) can lead to migraines, early disc degeneration, motor delays, spine curvature, or scoliosis, to name just a few. Sometimes even brain stem issues like Chiari malformation occur, where the lack of support causes the brain tissue to extend into the spinal canal, forcing it downward on the brain stem. Chronically tight muscles holding onto loose joints can cause musculoskeletal problems and, in some cases, persistent discomfort. Weakness, weariness, and certain movement issues can also arise, making daily activities difficult.

Symptoms of CCI can include headache or neck pain, weakness in the upper or lower extremities, sensory changes, clumsiness with frequent falls, uncertain gait, and fatigue. Those experiencing CCI report gastroesophageal disturbances and respiratory disorders, which manifest as sleep apnea, snoring, or history of frequent awakening. Most commonly reported are vestibular, auditory, or visual disturbance and bowel and/or bladder dysfunction. It is common for weather and environmental changes (e.g., cold weather and/or barometric changes) to induce an abnormal circulation response that can include profuse sweating, unrestful sleep, insomnia, frequent awakenings, and nightmares.

A common experience for people with EDS are a lot of unrelated and strange symptoms and variable disorders all masking the root cause of hypermobility. In my case, I was "diagnosed" with everything from Hashimoto's thyroiditis and alopecia to Sjögren's and celiac disease. I admittedly had a strange medical history, with multiple instances of adult chickenpox (five!), estrogen dominance syndrome, lifelong severe allergies and a history of Epstein-Barr virus. After many years of severe neck and shoulder pain, countless rounds of injections, nerve blocks, and painful dry needling to ease tight muscle spasms (and every other technique I could find), I was diagnosed correctly with craniocervical instability (CCI), atlantoaxial instability (AAI), and mild Chiari.

If you suspect you have instability in your neck, it is vital to get proper tests done to verify your range of motion and determine any instability in your joints. After months researching specialists across the US, I finally saw Dr. Fraser Henderson, an EDS specialist neurosurgeon outside of Washington, DC, who has contributed decades to the EDS community. He immediately ordered the proper tests for me to be accurately diagnosed.

There are two critical tests to determine craniocervical instability:

1. **An MRI scan of the cervical spine in an upright** (i.e., standing and not lying down face up horizontally called supine) position demonstrates the movement during neutral, flexion, and extension views as a dynamic image. This is where you must rotate your head downward and backward to see the degree of laxity in your hypermobility during flexion and extension variable measurements. They discovered my skull was sliding 5 mm off the back

of my skull and causing neurological symptoms such as imbalance, cognitive issues, pinched nerves, and cutting off arteries to my brain. It is necessary to have a standing MRI to pick up on the slippage and instability. Regular MRIs lying down don't correctly detect it.

2. A rotational CT scan (turning your head left and right and far as you can) shows precisely how far you can extend your head beyond the normal limits in millimeters. The rotational CT scan can detect atlantio-axial instability (AAI), by looking at the slippage of C1 off C2. If I'm getting too technical, think of it like a friend of mine explains it: "How you can be Regan from the horror film The Exorcist spinning your head around too far."

The proper imaging tests to determine CCI and AAI are simple, but it's hard to locate facilities that have the appropriate equipment or the technicians to properly read the results. There was only one facility in the entire DC Metro area for me. Understand you may need to travel to get the right tests done.

Combining these two tests can rule out neck instability and identify if there is hope in the form of surgery for recovery. Sometimes it can be the thing that helps your care team finally figure out what is wrong with you. It was in my case. You will know from the neurosurgeon at that point if you need surgery or should not run the risk. A home test for whether surgery will help is simply to wear a rigid neck brace (like the Alta Vista or Miami J collar) for two to four weeks around the clock. If your pain improves, you might be a good candidate for surgery.

Unfortunately, I learned that the neurosurgeon I needed to have surgery with did not accept medical insurance. Paying for a $150,000 procedure out of pocket plus hospital costs wasn't an option. I kept looking for options and got lucky. During a patient educational webinar sponsored by the Bobby Jones Chiari & Syringomyelia Foundation (CSF), I was introduced to Dr. Sunil Patel from Medical University at South Carolina (MUSC). I was able to get in within a few months and drove eight hours each way for a 30-minute appointment for another opinion on my need and possible approaches to surgery. He confirmed I needed a spinal fusion and suggested after his evaluation it span from my skull (occiput) to the C-3 vertebra.

Surgery and its aftereffects

Considering surgery of any type involves serious risks, but especially brain surgery, and you should weigh the pros and cons carefully. You need to work directly with your care team to determine the best decision for you. For me, I wanted to give it a chance to improve the quality of my life. When we were prepping for surgery, my loving and funny husband, John, asked the neurosurgeon to put a LED light in my skull for fun right before I was put under anesthesia to make me laugh. I needed it – I was a nervous wreck!

The best term to explain what happened next is "miraculous." I woke up at 5:00 a.m. the next morning in pain feeling like I had a metal LEGO in my head but a newfound sense of possibility. A new door opened as the blood flow returned to my brain. I felt great. According to many neurosurgeons and nurses at the hospital, I even looked good. I walked within a few hours and climbed the stairs the next day – a task I had not done well in a long while.

Many people I meet with potential CCI ask me about the recovery time and process. Of course it varies for everyone, but mine was a remarkable experience. I was on pain medications for less than a week and heavy-duty muscle relaxants for only a few weeks total. I had tried the experimental treatment gaining more popularity called prolotherapy on my neck to reduce the pain and muscle spasms. Prolotherapy is an injection of a saline and sugar-type fluid into your tissues to release the spasm muscles and increase healing.

In my case I was lucky enough to be showering within days, taking long walks, and occasionally bending my knees to stoop. Swallowing was hard at first but got better. With my neck fused, moving with confidence was difficult for a while, as I was cautious and afraid to damage my incision or affect the healing process or risk tethered cord damage. I have post-op ramifications, including the increased subluxing in my thoracic spine, progressive scoliosis, and ribs that pop out. I manage and monitor my spine as I may need future surgeries. But for now, I am pleased with my progress post-surgery. My recovery and physical therapy are still ongoing, and I continue to improve one year later.

Any dysfunction in your body combined with inflammation requires time to heal. I know my case is not the norm, and complications can erupt from bones not growing properly around the fusion and can require future fusions and other serious complications. I am very thankful to have enjoyed such a remarkable experience. But I believe it has a lot to do with attitude as well, which is what the rest of this book is about.

Not everything got better of course when you're dealing with EDS: my fatigue and chronic pain (though milder) still persist. Cognitive dysfunction and brain fog continue. The inability to rotate my head still makes driving challenging and unsafe. I had mild scoliosis in my back before, and as expected following the stabilization of one joint, the others started moving more. My spine looks like a model of the DNA helix, twirling around and swaying back and forth at more than a 20-degree angle at various points. I am likely to soon need another spinal surgery to stabilize lower facets from my cervical to thoracic spine junctures. Yet fifteen months post-surgery, I can gladly report I am better for the decision.

Choose to Assess, Act, or Affirm

- **Assess:** What, if anything, shocked you in this chapter?
- **Act:** What motivated you to act? What are your next steps? Write them down now.
- **Affirm:** "I am a friend to my body. I forgive my body and treat it with the same loving kindness I would like to receive."

Bibliography

"Mastocytosis." (2022). Cleveland Clinic. https://my.cleve landclinic.org/health/diseases/5908-mastocytosis.

Gensemer, C., Burks, R., Kautz, S., Judge, D. P., Lavallee, M., and Norris, R.A. (2020). "Hypermobile Ehlers-Danlos Syndromes: Complex Phenotypes, Challenging Diagnoses, and Poorly Understood Causes." *Dev Dyn.* 250(3): 318–344. doi: 10.1002/dvdy.220. Epub 2020 Aug 17. PMID: 32629534.

Mayo Clinic. (2020). "Prolotherapy: Solution to Low Back Pain?" https://www.mayoclinic.org/prolotherapy/expert-answers/faq-20058347.

"Postural Orthostatic Tachycardia Syndrome (POTS): State of the Science, Clinical Care, and Research," National Heart, Lung, and Blood Institute, July 29, 2019. https://www.nhlbi.nih.gov/events/2019/postural-ortho static-tachycardia-syndrome-pots-state-science-clinical-care-and-research#:~:text=Many%20POTS%20special-ists%20have%20lengthy,for%20POTS%2Drelated%20 medical%20care.

Wang, E., Ganti, T., Vaou, E., and Hohler, A. (2021). "The Relationship between Mast Cell Activation Syndrome, Postural Tachycardia Syndrome, and Ehlers-Danlos Syndrome." *Allergy Asthma Proc.* 42(3): 243–246. doi: 10.2500/aap.2021.42.210022. PMID: 33980338.

NOTES

PART II

COPING WITH EDS

They say all girls love diamonds for their beauty, and certainly they are. But I have a different perspective. I see diamonds as unique and rare objects formed from a great deal of pressure and crushing stress. Sounds a bit like facing a chronic invisible illness, huh?

Chronic illness can crush you into a new form as well. If you are struggling with hEDS, you are undoubtedly feeling the pressure and even feeling crushed by the process of trying to get help and find knowledgeable care team members and lifestyle solutions to enhance your quality of life. Many people think the result of an EDS diagnosis is something awful, but what I hope to impart in this book is the realization that as a result of EDS you are unique, you are enough, and should think of yourself as a rare and beautiful diamond. You are multifaceted and formed by sometimes painful processes and occasionally have to chip away to find the real you. I sometimes think of myself as flawsome – flawed and awesome combined!

Facing your fears and the vulnerability it can bring is as hard as I would imagine a diamond formed in the Earth's crust is. As rare as a zebra sighting in the wild. But zebras can shine through hard work and effort – that's why a group of zebras is called a "dazzle." That's why developing coping skills is so important. Fellow zebras, prepare to dazzle the world with our rare brilliance – just like a diamond.

CHAPTER 4

DEALING WITH PAIN

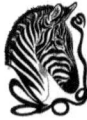

*Shame does not have to silence us unless we let it.
Whether you experienced something traumatic or felt
shame about not having it all together, speak up.
Shame cannot exist if you have empathy, a voice,
and acceptance. We all experience shame, for different reasons, at different times. It's okay. There's no
shame in being you. Please re-read that again and
again. You are not your worst decision. No matter
what you've done, you deserve love, empathy, and
understanding. And you are never alone.*

– Lauren Darlington

The pain of a broken bone or burst appendix is not easy
to deal with, but at least the end is in sight. As soon as

the bone or abdomen heals, you will be back to normal. That is not true for chronic conditions such as high blood pressure, heart failure, diabetes, arthritis, osteoporosis, or other harmful disorders such as EDS. Unlike acute diagnoses such as the flu, and sometimes even the tragedy of a cancer diagnosis where a predictable course of treatment exists, with a chronic illness there is no cure in sight, and they usually last a lifetime. You'll have to learn to live with a continuous day-to-day situation, responding to rapidly changing symptoms and problems.

Chronic illness also requires ongoing medical care and brings difficulties doing the things you need to do every day. These behaviors (called "activities of daily living" by the medical community) can include simple personal things such as using the toilet and getting dressed. Not being able to fully care for yourself is life-altering. These difficulties can affect your family and your relationships with those who care about you. Many people are left without loved ones to help care for them in their times of need. You feel very alone, even ashamed, and dismissed with an invisible illness that others typically cannot see (it might be a little easier if we looked sick!). It is hard for others to understand what we go through.

Most people go through stages in learning to cope with a chronic illness. These go alongside the stages of grief.

1. **Reaction/shock: The first stage involves facing your initial feelings about your new health**

condition. Some people feel vulnerable, confused, and worried about their health and the future. Others feel sad or disappointed in their bodies. For some, the situation seems unfair, causing them to feel angry at themselves and those they love. These feelings are the beginning of the process. I did not handle the early stages well at all. It caused me to disconnect from my family and even my child as they found me unpleasant to be around. Everyone's reaction to chronic illness in themselves or a loved one can be different, but they're all completely normal. Try to give yourself grace.

2. **Becoming more aware: The second stage in the process is actively learning everything you can about your disease.** Most people living with a long-term or incurable illness find that knowledge is power. The more they find out about their condition, the more they feel in control and the less frightening it is. The best way to learn about your condition and put yourself in power is to ask questions, learn, and design potential solutions with your care team.

3. **Finding acceptance: The third stage in coping with a chronic illness is all about taking it in stride.** I do not mean giving up but finding peace with it. At this stage, people feel more comfortable with their treatments and the tools (such as inhalers or mobility aids) they need to use to live

everyday life. When the condition is first diagnosed people may feel a range of emotions. Fear sets in, and we make the early mistake of simply googling the disease. However, after working with doctors and understanding more about their condition, that person will grow to be more practiced at monitoring and managing their feelings. Over time, much like a diabetic adjusts to taking insulin and required dietary changes, it becomes second nature, and the steps involved are similar to daily care like teeth brushing or showering.

4. **Allowing yourself to adapt:** Hopefully, someday you learn to cope. There's no definite time limit on the coping process. Everybody's process of coming to terms with and accepting a chronic illness varies. In fact, most people will find that emotions surface at all stages in the grief process. Even if treatments go well, it's natural to feel sad or worried from time to time. Recognizing and being aware of these emotions as they surface is all part of the process. Most importantly, to start coping, you must approach it with a success mindset. Fear is just a feeling you can learn to cope with. Just like you've learned to cope with your pain. Fear can paralyze you and keep you stuck physically, mentally, and emotionally. Don't let it. Try to reframe how you think about fear as an acronym: **F**ace **E**verything **A**nd **R**ise.

Developing coping skills

Adjusting to living with a chronic illness takes time, patience, and support — and a willingness to learn and participate. People who deal with unexpected challenges often find an inner resilience they might not have known was there before. Many say that they learn more about themselves by dealing with these challenges and feel they grow stronger and more self-aware than they would if they'd never faced any other particular challenge. People living with chronic illnesses find that when they take an active role in taking care of their bodies, they grow to understand and appreciate their strengths — and adapt to their weaknesses — as never before.

When pain is present in the body, it's normal to experience a fear-based response in the brain. Most people do not realize that this holds true in reverse as well: When fear is present in the brain, it is natural to feel it in the body. How astonishing would it be if you had some control over the pain and suffering? I believe we can change our thinking and daily habits to live better. We have to break the cycle to survive and thrive with EDS or any chronic illness.

In chronic pain, fear and pain fuel each other. They put the mind in a downward spiral of anxiety. They can make the experience of pain much worse. It makes it too easy for our caveman autonomic nervous systems and bodies to activate our fight-or-flight system. When you learn how to reduce the fear, you also may be able to decrease mental anxiety and improve your daily life, reduce the physical intensity of your symptoms, and often reduce the frequency of your flare-ups. That means you can enjoy activities that bring you joy that you might be avoiding because of fear. Neuroscience proves this change in your brain is possible.

The most important step you can take is to seek help as soon as you feel like you need help, which is often early on. Speak up to your doctors and keep a journal of your issues where you try to describe the pain sensations and rate it on a scale of 1–10. Taking action early will help you understand and deal with the many effects of a chronic illness as they become more predictable. It is imperative to learn to manage pain, and that will help you maintain a positive outlook on life. Identify strategies that can help you regain a sense of control and improve your quality of life – something everyone deserves. If you're suffering from depression, your medical provider may prescribe medications to help regulate your mood and make you feel better. But there are other things you can do on your own that will help. This book aims to share such helpful tips, such as the ones described here that have helped me climb out of the despair of chronic illness.

The warning light is on

Pain is a simple system doing its job – the body's warning light coming on signaling that something is not right. It should not be ignored. When painful symptoms first arise, patients and their care team work together to see if they can identify and address the underlying cause, which could be unstable joints or a number of other causes. Sometimes there is no precise medical or surgical cure for many conditions and injuries, and without an identifiable cause, patients may be diagnosed with chronic pain. Treatment goals will then shift from resolving the pain to reducing and/or managing it.

Pain is considered chronic when it persists for three to six months or more. But for some patients, chronic pain can last for years or even a lifetime.

Chronic pain facts according to the US Pain Foundation:

- Chronic pain affects 50 million American adults, or 20% of the population;
- Chronic pain is associated with reduced quality of life and a higher incidence of depression, anxiety, and suicidal ideation;
- Pain is the number one reason Americans access the health care system;
- Pain is the leading cause of long-term disability in the United States;
- The United States spends approximately $600 billion each year on chronic pain in terms of medical costs, disability payments, and lost productivity;
- Veterinary students spent seven times as many education hours focused on pain management as medical students;

- There is only one board-certified pain specialist for every 10,000 people with severe pain;

- The National Institutes of Health dedicates approximately 2% of its funding to pain research, a miniscule amount relative to its societal burden;

- Studies have shown that minority groups and marginalized populations are more likely to receive suboptimal care.

Because each person with pain is unique, it can be challenging to manage pain effectively and often takes a trial-and-error approach to find solutions that suit you. Typically, successful pain management requires finding a combination of multidisciplinary, multimodal therapies that reduce pain enough to improve quality of life and increase function. These therapies should include psychosocial strategies that address the whole person, including their emotional and mental health. While it's easy to get frustrated when a particular therapy option doesn't work, don't give up. Most likely, something else will help—you must keep searching for answers.

Once you receive a chronic pain diagnosis or have lived with pain for more than three months, it's a good idea to get connected with a pain specialist. While clinicians in specialties such as neurology and orthopedics may offer some pain management options, it's essential to have someone on your team who is an expert in pain itself if you have hEDS. It is also common to have nerve-related pain and neuropathy as a result. This requires particular doctor-supervised administration of treatments for nerve pain.

ABOUT CHRONIC INFLAMMATION

Harvard Medical puts out insights on how chronic inflammation can develop in many ways. One possibility is that a threat remains because the body can't rid itself of the offending substance, be it an infectious organism, an irritant, or a chemical toxin. The immune system is pretty good at eliminating foreign invaders, but sometimes pathogens resist even our best defenses and hide in the tissues, provoking the inflammatory response again and again. Another possible scenario is that the immune system goes into threat mode when no true threat exists, as in an autoimmune disorder. It can react against the joints, intestines, or other organs and tissues as if they were dangerous. As the inflammatory response continues, it damages the body instead of healing it.

The signs of chronic inflammation are not as obvious as those of acute inflammation. No sharp twinge of pain as when you cut yourself, no swelling or redness will you see to alert you to a problem. Chronic inflammation can be widespread or more localized to specific areas of the body. Therefore, symptoms can vary considerably, such as:

- Fatigue and lack of energy;
- Depression and/or anxiety;

- Muscle aches and joint pain;
- Constipation, diarrhea, and other gastrointestinal complaints;
- Changes in weight or appetite;
- Headaches;
- A fuzzy mental state (brain fog).

If you can get to a pain clinic or center, find one that emphasizes multidisciplinary care. A good indicator is when the center employs a range of specialists in addition to traditional pain doctors—for example, psychologists, clinical social workers, sleep medicine experts, nutritionists, and/or physical therapists.

The precise cause of pain in hypermobility syndromes is not clear, and each of us responds differently to various techniques to manage pain. Your doctor will be able to help you decide which to try based on your symptoms and any contraindications involved. While an experienced pain specialist will have a lot of suggestions for treatment, it's imperative to educate yourself on the various strategies and techniques available for pain relief. Keep in mind, too, that researchers are always making headway in discovering new treatments.

Common types of pain in hypermobile EDS

Long-term or chronic pain in hEDS typically appears early as a first symptom, is very common, and may be severe and unmanageable for some. According to the Ehlers-Danlos Society, some of the common causes and contributors to chronic pain include joints coming out of position (subluxing), previous surgery (often done to treat pain), muscle weakness and atrophy, improper hypermobile movement in the neck and back, or issues with a sense of joint position (proprioception). The pain those with hEDS experience comes in different forms—injuries, fatigue, and chronic persistent pain.

Hypermobile people can often get injured from over-extending joints, falls, mishaps, exercise, sports, and more. Obviously, going to urgent care or the ER can be necessary sometimes. Home management of acute and immediate pain is essential and usually done best with alternating ice and heat therapies. Ice should be applied first to reduce any swelling or inflammation. It's good for acute pain and short-term relief and should be used for about 20 minutes on, then 20 minutes off. Heat can be applied once it has calmed down to increase the blood flow to the area. Heat is used alternatively to loosen up the muscles, but it can increase inflammation, so use it cautiously and check with your care providers on which to use for your situation. You should get quality ice packs and heat packs because you'll be using them regularly. Long story short: The tried and true acronym RICE works—rest, ice, compression, and elevation.

Because the tendons and ligaments of someone with hEDS are so much stretchier than usual, the body must work much harder to perform tasks, such as sitting, standing, and walking. This causes tissues to become fatigued much more quickly than a healthy person's body would. This means those with hEDS can struggle to perform relatively simple tasks and must be careful not to do too much. I have found it particularly difficult to learn what I can and can't do and learn to pace myself. It is tough to say no to activities you would love to do but that you know would either not be good for you or have a lasting detrimental effect. The cycle of overdoing it can lead to me being confined to bed for days to recover. In addition to physical fatigue, cognitive dysfunction occurs, including memory loss, difficulty thinking and concentrating, and sleep problems.

The pain people with EDS feel can present very differently. Many people feel like everything hurts, while others describe acute pain in specific parts of the body such as the head, stomach, groin, shoulder, neck, or jaw. When your bones are not stabilized, your muscles are working overtime to compensate for holding things in place and, at a minimum, are very tight and painful. Many people with EDS experience neuropathic pain, caused by damage to the various levels of the nervous system—the spinal cord, brain, and peripheral nerves. Like many people with hEDS, I struggle daily with various types of chronic pain, including joint pain, muscle pain (due to chronic tightness and due to spasms), nerve pain, and headaches. This pain often cannot be controlled with medication alone and is something I am learning to cope with constantly.

Flare-ups can happen when your pain is not properly treated or managed consistently, or you have overdone it. During a flare up, pain suddenly worsens and may last a short time or a few days or weeks. Unfortunately, learning how to manage and even predict your flare-ups is a skill you will learn the hard way. It is very important to listen to your body. It can be helpful to create a pain action plan for you and those who care for you to have access to during flare-ups. Try to remind yourself the flare is probably temporary. Tools such as relaxation, distractions, rest, or maybe gentle movement with good hydration can help heal your tissues faster.

CREATE A PAIN MANAGEMENT ACTION PLAN

Gwenn Herman of the US Pain Foundation shared her insights including her Pain Action Plan described fully in her book, *Making the Invisible Visible: Chronic Pain Manual for Health Care Providers*. The plan she suggests is that people should recognize and write down how they experience pain and what to do about when they experience a flare. It can also help their family who is watching them suffer.

The pain action plan breaks down into four Rs: **R**ecognize, **R**espond, **R**ecruit, and **R**evise.

1. **Recognize** helps you determine what your warning signs or triggers are—both physically

and mentally—and to write them down. Like flashing lights or a particular sound or sensation.

2. **Respond** is to identify and write down how you respond to the symptoms.

3. **Recruiting** is deciding and capturing methods of how and what you need to deal with your pain. For example, what specific action do you usually use like ice/heat, medications, or rest. The action plan written down is not only for you but for your family members and significant others. This allows your brain to have a go-to list for you and others of how to help in a flare.

4. **Revise** is reevaluating the plan when you're not in a flare so you and others have a plan in writing to best support you in those moments of extreme pain when you don't always think or react at your best.

Treating pain

Medications may be used depending on the type of pain, such as pain from inflammation, or for immediate relief from severe pain. Harvard Health says analgesics (painkillers) are the most common pain remedy. Acetaminophen (Tylenol and other brand names) interferes with pain messages, while aspirin and ibuprofen (Advil, Motrin, and others) do that as well as reduce inflammation, swelling, and irritation that can worsen the pain. Nonsteroidal anti-inflammatory drugs (NSAIDs) can be helpful when there's an acute injury, such as a pulled ligament, subluxation, or dislocation, and where the tissues have become inflamed and swollen. Rheumatologists often suggest over-the-counter (OTC) anti-inflammatory drugs such as ibuprofen or acetaminophen to treat mild pain. These can be helpful as they are easily accessible and affordable. Follow instructions and don't take NSAIDs for too long because they can cause stomach pain and ulcers, high blood pressure, kidney problems, and trigger an attack in those who are asthmatic.

Topical pain relievers (such as lidocaine patches, IcyHot, Aspercreme, Tiger Balm, or BenGay) may lessen pain by numbing the area, reducing inflammation, or causing a form of skin irritation that distracts the brain from focusing on pain. Medications such as gabapentin or Lyrica (pregabalin) are prescribed to try and control either local nerve pain or widespread pain where the body is susceptible to touch. Some EDS patients swear by the help they receive from stimulants to increase their energy and reduce fatigue. Many use the commonly prescribed drug Adderall. I understand many get relief from fatigue-reducing prescriptions such as Provigil or its less expensive generic equivalent. Be aware of the increase in anxiety it can cause.

Narcotic pain relievers, such as morphine, codeine, and opioids, are some of the most powerful pain medications on the market. These usually are reserved for the most intense pain; they are highly addictive and can cause constipation as well as other serious side effects. I am personally very wary of addictive narcotic pain medications such as OxyContin. If you aren't sure about what opioids can potentially do to your life, binge-watch the Netflix series *Dopesick* for a rude yet sad awakening. Also be aware that asking for opiates can wind up with you being labeled with "drug-seeking" behavior by your providers. Many people cannot get through the day without them while the medical community is torn on the use of opioids for regular pain management.

Other drugs such as anesthetics, antidepressants, anticonvulsants, and corticosteroids may work against certain types of pain. Muscle relaxers can be tricky for hypermobile people, whose muscles are spending all their energy holding us together. If you allow that tightness to relax, it can cause more problems. I have been helped by muscle relaxers occasionally only in low doses on an as-needed basis. Sometimes medications are injected directly into the region of pain or near a nerve to interrupt the pain signal, including steroids or local anesthetics. For very severe pain episodes, hydrocortisone injections may be necessary; lidocaine can be helpful when joints misalign, for spastic muscles, gum pain, and in severe cases of painful intercourse. Overall, the pain management approach should focus on treating the root cause (such as joints coming out of position) and lowering the pain sensation overall.

Many people metabolize pain and other medications at abnormal rates. To help your doctor determine what is best for you, pharmaco-genetic testing may be helpful. Some drugs used for treating pain, such as opioids or NSAIDs (ibuprofen, naproxen), can be harmful over long periods or in EDS patients with mast cell activation syndrome. Drugs for nerve pain may not be suitable in hEDS because of their effect on bodily functions already severely affected. Some medicines or combinations of drugs may improve uncontrolled muscle contractions, pain, and tiredness. Be careful and consult a physician when considering taking medicine.

Practitioners who treat pain include primary care providers, physiatrists, osteopaths, physical therapists, neurologists, surgeons, anesthesiologists, and pain management specialists, so it's essential to find out the source of the pain and how best to treat it. Pain management practitioners can help patients learn skills

DR. ERIC SINGMAN'S ADVICE ON MIGRAINE PAIN

"Many EDS patients suffer from migraines. I suggest they keep a diary and log in the journal how often and when they're getting headaches and the surrounding circumstances. I try to help them educate themselves to be able to go on an anti-migraine diet. That means no wine, no caffeine, no hard cheeses, etc. I also suggest that they take supplements including magnesium, CoQ10, and B vitamins. It has been shown to elevate your migraine threshold and reduce the duration and frequency of migraines." Read the interview with Dr. Singman in the Appendix.

needed to improve their quality of life despite their pain, rather than reducing their pain. This approach focuses on the total person. In many cases, the pain will be treated by more than one specialist and often in more than one modality or method.

Pain specialists use several alternative treatments in addition to or instead of pain medication. One place to start is with lifestyle changes, including dietary changes to include less inflammatory foods such as sugar, alcohol, or gluten, plus the addition of mild, regular exercise and meditation. Other standard methods of pain management often include various types of support pillows and cushions to ease discomfort while sitting or lying and/or compression clothing that helps with positional sensing and support braces. I've gotten the best relief and the best night's sleep from a pillow that's adjustable by measuring the amount of water to raise or lower the density inside, called a Medipillow. Even the use of ice and heat can modify pain. I was amazed when my massage therapist recommended I put a bag of frozen brussels sprouts on the base of my skull and neck to ease pain. The hard frozen vegetables had the cooling and anti-inflammatory effect that aided in pain relief.

Joint protection is a vital aspect of managing hypermobility, as exaggerated movements create pain and risk injury. The aim is to reduce strain on the joints by stabilizing and spreading the load over several joints, such as using both legs when lifting or using braces. Overcompensating on one side of your body can also lead to more pain. Splinting, bracing, taping, compression wear, and custom-made orthotics, including mouthguards for TMJ, are all methods used to manage joint hypermobility.

Physiotherapy is also widely considered among the most beneficial methods of managing hEDS. This type of therapy is provided by a trained specialist involving manual therapy, prescribed home exercises, and education. Treatment goals include helping to keep joints and muscles strong and moving, easing pain, and keeping the patient as mobile as possible. Physiotherapy may include work on proprioception, strength, balance, relaxing tight muscles, and building endurance. Depending on a patient's presentation of symptoms, treatment might focus on the musculoskeletal system, nerves, heart, blood vessels, lungs, or a combination of these systems.

In his *Joint Hypermobility Handbook* (2010), Dr. Brad Tinkle shares that increasing muscle strength promotes joint stability and, together with postural awareness and correction, is the starting point for improving many symptoms. He reminds us that hypermobile EDS is a genetic condition of the collagen meaning while muscle strength can compensate to some degree, it may never create the kind of stability that is inherently present for non-hypermobile.

Physical therapy can help with pain management through improving stability, strength, and proprioception, which is the loss of sense of joint position and can be an essential factor in hEDS-related chronic pain.

Some providers also often use a transcutaneous electrical nerve stimulation (TENS) device to help redirect your nerve pain by resetting the signals. Other pain specialists can perform a procedure called a radio frequency ablation (RFA) to stop nerve pinching severe pain. These cauterize the nerve endings and can resolve pain for several months providing longer-lasting relief. I had several successful nerve ablation treatments on my neck before they became ineffective.

Many people with hEDS have had pain relief and improved stability with prolotherapy or platelet rich plasma (PRP). PRP and prolotherapy get mixed reviews—I tried prolotherapy in my neck for pain and muscle spasms, which made me significantly worse, but others I know have experienced pain relief success. And of course many EDSers struggle to decide whether they should have surgery to repair damaged joints (as described in Chapter 3). Talk to your doctor and get educated about your options.

Other useful aids for pain include magnets, splints, grip pens and special cooking utensils, ergonomic keyboards, wedges, mobility aids, mattresses and shock-absorbing insoles, all of which can help reduce pain and aid in independent living. Some improvements can be yielded from braces or splints to prevent joint mobility (discussed in a later chapter).

You can also learn more about the US Pain Foundation's best resources for chronic pain at www.uspainfoundation. org/pain/treatment. The following are their tips for treatment (shared with permission):

- **Start small:** If your pain levels allow it, start with low-risk, noninvasive treatment options, like physical therapy and cognitive behavioral therapy, before moving to more serious interventions. While medications, injections, and surgeries can be vital components of pain management, they come with risks and side effects. Especially when it comes to invasive procedures, consider getting a second opinion.

- **Do your homework:** Use the internet or your local library to research your condition and evidence-based treatments. Try to verify that the information is reliable; government agencies, patient-led organizations, and well-known sites. Educating yourself is especially important if your condition is rare—even with the best intentions, your doctor may not have the time or resources to research the nuances of your disease.

- **Maximize your doctors' visits:** Bring a list of questions, and think carefully about your goals for your appointment. Don't be afraid to advocate for yourself and your needs. If possible, ask a family member or friend to come with you. They can help support you, and having a second pair of ears to absorb all the information from your doctor can be helpful.

- **Stay organized:** Dealing with complex health issues can be a part- or even full-time job in and of itself. To help juggle your various appointments, test results, therapy options, and insurance issues consider starting a binder or folder with everything in one place. Remember, too, that you have the right to request your medical records and test results from any provider you see.

- **Prioritize your mental health**: Many people with pain are so busy managing their physical health that they forget to take care of themselves emotionally. But chronic pain can affect your mood and stress levels, and likewise, your mood and stress levels can affect your chronic pain. Talk to your care provider about ways to mitigate the emotional impact of pain, like connecting with a support group or experienced counselor.

- **Be the squeaky wheel:** If your insurance company denies a treatment option or says a specialist is not in-network, don't give up! Ask your clinician to help you appeal the decision, or appeal it yourself. In addition, many states have health advocacy offices that can help with insurance issues. Try reaching out to them for assistance if your appeal is unsuccessful.

Medical cannabis and CBD

Clinical research suggests that cannabis can help with pain relief, nausea, appetite, seizures, mood, and sleep. Even though medical cannabis can be an effective treatment option for people with pain, its use has long been stigmatized by society, resulting in many misunderstandings. This is a sensitive subject for many people whether you are pro or con. I share a few well-founded facts from the pain-related community, and you can do your own research and draw your own conclusions for your situation on if cannabis is suitable for your pain.

It is helpful to go over a glossary of commonly used terms relative to cannabis use.

- *Cannabis* refers to the part of the plant *Cannabis sativa* L, which has been cultivated by humans for thousands of years, provides a variety of uses including hemp.

- *Marijuana* is the flowering top of the cannabis plant used for ceremonial, medicinal, or other purposes for thousands of years.

- *Endocannabinoid* system is the regulatory system in the human body that deals with memory, hunger, emotion, stress, and immune function.

- *Phytocannabinoid* is a cannabinoid produced in nature by the cannabis plant.

- *THC* is the most well-known phytocannabinoid. It is medicinal as well as a tool for relaxation. Uses include treatment for pain, nausea, insomnia, and more.

- *CBD* is another phytocannabinoid. CBD is highly medicinal and can assist with seizure control, neuroprotectant, anti-inflammatory issues, and more.

Medical cannabis is made of two components: THC, which causes the mental effects associated with feeling high, and CBD, which produces bodily effects. Various strains of cannabis have different ratios of THC and CBD, which means that not all strains create a high feeling. There are two main categories of medical cannabis strains: indica and sativa. The indica strains have higher CBD and lower THC counts. They can help with increased mental and muscle relaxation, decreased nausea and acute pain, and increased appetite and dopamine. Indica is typically preferred for nighttime use. Meanwhile, sativa strains have lower CBD and higher THC counts. They can help with anxiety and depression, chronic pain, and increased focus and serotonin. Sativa is usually preferred for daytime use.

Like with any medication, various types affect people differently, depending on how much you use and your specific body chemistry. Other factors that influence the effect include method of consumption, which includes smoking, pills, tinctures, topicals, patches, oils, and edibles, as well as mindset or mood.

In most US states that allow medical marijuana, a doctor would need to sign a form (not a prescription) identifying and confirming you have a qualifying condition. Typically, you would then use this documentation to apply for a medical cannabis card from your state if permitted by state law. Check out this website to find out the laws in your state: www.safeaccessnow.org.

The co-director for cannabis advocacy at the US Pain Foundation is Ellen Lenox Smith, who happens to suffer from EDS and previously spent years in a wheelchair. In her case, she lost the ability to metabolize medicine and turned to cannabis as an alternative. She has a wealth of knowledge about medical marijuana and is passionate about how it helped her. You can contact her at ellen@uspainfoundation.org. She graciously shared her homemade cannabis oil recipe below (reproduced with permission).

ELLEN'S HOMEMADE CANNABIS OIL RECIPE

Oil is obviously safer for your lungs because you are not smoking it. It's also easier to store and travel with (be sure you carry your RX).

1. Grind up the product in a coffee bean grinder or mixer.
2. Heat up 1 cup of extra virgin olive oil (or oil of choice), being careful to get it hot but not boiling.
3. Measure 10 Tbs of the ground product per 1 cup of oil.
4. Spread the product over the oil and listen for sizzling sounds (like Alka Seltzer dropped in water) as it's released into the oil. Sprinkle any remaining product over the oil and turn the heat off.
5. Allow the mixture to cool.
6. Strain the oil into a plastic or glass container for storage (away from the sun).

You can double or triple the recipe to make a larger batch—just maintain the 10 Tbs ground product to one cup oil ratio. Or if you want it even easier, try buying a MagicalButter machine (https://magicalbutter.com/) that allows you to put the ingredients together, plug it in and let it make the oil for you.

How to Use the Oil

Remember that when ingesting the oil you must allow time for it to be absorbed before you get pain relief. When first taken this way, it may take up to a full hour to feel the changes. Eventually, it may take less time. It's important to figure out when you will need relief so you are sure to get it into your system before the pain sets in.

Dosage Guidance to Start

Start with a low dose (1/4 tsp mixed with some food like a little applesauce or yogurt) to introduce this to your body slowly. Try taking one hour before your nightly sleep.

The goal is to eventually sleep through the night and not wake up groggy. Each night add 1/4 tsp more until you have slept the night but not woken up groggy in the morning. If that sensation happens, don't panic. It will wear off throughout the morning and reminds you to not take that dose again but decrease it.

Other alternative pain interventions

Usually the first line of treatment is typically pain medication. But while these medications may work for some people, in others, the side effects—ranging from nausea to heart complications—may outweigh the relief. Some patients explore options beyond pharmaceuticals alone or in tandem with traditional medicine; there are several options to consider, including acupuncture, chiropractic, vitamin or herbal supplements, and therapy. Whatever approach you choose, it's vital to remember that there is no one-size-fits-all approach to pain management.

Complementary therapy options can be an excellent place to start because they are less invasive and come with fewer risks but are not usually covered by insurance. Keep an open mind and talk with your provider about the different options available.

Acupuncture is standard in Chinese medicine and involves inserting thin, tiny needles into specific points of the body. Traditional Chinese practitioners believe acupuncture balances the flow of energy or life force known as qi, or chi. Western practitioners see it as a way to stimulate nerves and muscles to promote pain relief and healing. Many practitioners are now beginning to recognize the potential benefits of acupuncture.

A chiropractor's main objective is to realign and manipulate the spine and neck in a way that relieves pain, promotes healing, and improves overall function. There are many different styles of chiropractic care, and chiropractors use a wide range of strategies, techniques, and products as part of treatment. It's crucial to find a reputable, experienced practitioner and to be sure to understand the risks and benefits in advance of treatment as well as contraindications for hypermobility.

Another therapy I use regularly is floating. It's when you go to a float therapy studio where they have the giant Epsom salt pods that you float in like a specialized bath experience. It's typically for 60 minutes. The Epsom salt in the water releases magnesium into your system and eases your muscle pain and fatigue, and you will literally walk out of there feeling better. I have found over time that I feel better when I maintain a regular monthly routine. If you can't find a place to do floating, just soaking in an Epsom salts bath at home does wonders. Add two large cups of Epsom salts in the tub and soak for 10–20 minutes. You might also consider adding essential oils such as lavender to calm or orange to energize and apply topical magnesium oil to your skin after the bath.

There are an overwhelming number and array of vitamin, herbal or plant-based supplements to explore for pain relief. In some cases, these supplements may support overall well-being, which can, in turn, help reduce pain. In some instances, supplements may provide more direct relief by reducing inflammation or improving joint health. Examples of vitamin supplements include B vitamins, which support nerve health, and Vitamin C and D for bone health. An herbal or plant-based example would consist of turmeric or aloe vera. I also take serrapeptase supplements for pain management.

Counseling and therapy, including cognitive behavioral therapy (CBT), may be helpful when pain is difficult to control and shown to be beneficial in managing chronic pain and other physical health problems. CBT is similar to talk therapy that combines examining the things patients think cognitively and do behaviorally. This helps patients consider how thoughts and actions may be affecting the pain and other symptoms they experience. Instead of being thought of in purely physical terms, it's now widely recognized that persistent pain is made up of both physical and psychological factors. Health care professionals recognize this and suggest that chronic pain patients benefit from CBT from a trained licensed professional. Note that EDS patients often encounter practitioners who express skepticism that their pain is real.

Everyone experiences pain differently. Emotional influences such as whether or not you feel supported and understood, your personal life circumstances, or how tired or happy you are at the time do not cause physical pain, but they can certainly influence it. How you cope can also depend on your previous experiences, your beliefs about pain, and how you feel about yourself and your self-management skills.

Many doctors recommend a "toolbox" approach to pain management. Dr. Clair Francomano, world-renowned EDS medical expert, believes that "medications can take care of 20% of your pain relief. Then you use your TENS unit for another 10% reduction. Maybe a topical analgesic like Tiger Balm on your painful joints brings another 5% of pain relief. You can pull out your heat pad for another 5% of pain relief. Then you decide upon a warm soak with Epsom salts for another 10% pain relief. Deep breathing and some physiotherapy exercises combine for another 10%. And then you watch a great movie to distract you for another 15% of pain relief, so now you have about 75% of your pain managed effectively." Overall, the best pain treatment is what works for you and your body. Everyone's body responds differently. Try different things until you find something that you can live with.

The management of the often severe, changing, and debilitating pain in patients with hEDS is currently just not good enough. Commonly used pain medications do not help treat all patients, probably because the cause of pain is different. There is no one-size-fits-all solution yet. Many pain medications have disadvantages, including addiction, dependence, and destruction of the body's systems over time.

I encourage you to find a pain management specialist who understands EDS. If you see a pain management specialist, review the available options and do your homework before you agree to any treatment plan.

Always seek advice from your doctor concerning any recommendations before you try them. They are trained to check the most current information provided on the procedures or the manufacturer of each product to be administered and to verify the recommended dose and formula, the methods and duration, and contraindications.

Choose to Assess, Act, or Affirm

- **Assess:** Did you learn any new methods or ideas to help you cope with pain?
- **Act:** Try visual imagery and/or distraction to ease your pain. Imagery involves concentrating on mental

pictures of pleasant scenes or events or mentally repeating positive words or phrases to reduce pain. Google "guided imagery" for ideas. Distraction techniques focus attention away from harmful or painful images to positive mental thoughts. This technique may include simple activities, such as watching television or a favorite movie, reading a book or listening to a book on tape, listening to music, or talking to a friend.

- **Affirm:** "I'm listening and learning from my pain."

Bibliography

Criscione, Michael. (2021). "Chronic Pain: The Impact on 50 Million Americans." Healthline. https://www.healthline.com/health-news/chronic-pain-the-impact-on-the-50-million-americans-who-have-it.

The Ehlers Danlos Society. (2017). "Pain Management in the Ehlers-Danlos Syndromes." https://www.ehlers-danlos.com/pdf/2017-FINAL-AJMG-PDFs/Chopra_et_al-2017-American_Journal_of_Medical_Genetics_Part_C-_Seminars_in_Medical_Genetics.pdf.

Dahlhamer, J. et al. (2018). "Prevalence of Chronic Pain and High-Impact Chronic Pain Among Adults." *MMWR Morb Mortal Wkly Rep*, 67:1001–1006. https://www.cdc.gov/mmwr/volumes/67/wr/mm6736a2.htm.

US Pain Foundation. (2021). "Treatment." https://uspainfoundation.org/pain/treatment/.

NOTES

CHAPTER 5

NAVIGATING THE MEDICAL SYSTEM

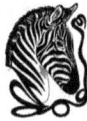

The next time you face a challenging situation, hit your internal pause button, breathe, and survey the situation. Don't panic. Ask yourself, what can I do right now? What is the number one priority? Accept that what has happened, happened. Don't beat yourself up for what you didn't do. Drop resistance and fighting what is, and instead focus on what you can do now. Focus on what's good in the situation. Ask yourself, what are the lessons to be learned from this? And make a gratitude list as fast as possible. Think about the good things that came from the events rather than constantly repeating a negative story to others. Integrate the lessons, let it go, and move on.

—**Polly Green**

One of the critical aspects of successfully managing hEDS is coming to terms with and understanding the fact that you must see a multitude of different types of medical providers and specialists who evaluate and treat you for bodily systems they know in a silo. As a result, American medical systems fail with respect to identifying interlocking health issues and caring for us holistically. That is definitely the case for a chronic connective tissue disorder such as EDS. Because connective tissues include your skin, veins, muscles, and ligaments, it quite literally affects *everywhere in your body.* Not everyone will have symptoms in all areas and resulting pain or problems, but seeing the connection and properly diagnosing the resulting array of symptoms are quite elusive to diagnose by untrained medical professionals.

I find myself oftentimes having to deliver difficult news on the phone to potential clients who suspect they might have hypermobility and asked, "Where can I go see an EDS doctor and get the procedure to fix this?" Given the disparity of specialists and because EDS affects multiple bodily functions and systems, there are currently no specialists nor any one procedure or test for hypermobility to evaluate you holistically and see the commonality of issues. What's worse is the fact that those doctors that do have a specialty touching on EDS are often overwhelmed by patients, and their waiting lists can literally be months or even years long.

Dr. Sunil Patel, one of my doctors and an expert hEDS neurosurgeon at MUSC, explained this very clearly. "EDS is a very complex set of disorders that are not going to be managed by one specialist or another. It's going to require the engagement of physical therapists, neurosurgeons, orthopedic surgeons, cardiologists, gastroenterologists, immunologists, rheumatologists, etc., who come together hopefully to early diagnose these patients, and then co-manage these patients to help them achieve a more functional life." While medical mysteries on television are invariably solved in an hour, in reality it really takes a village and a lot of patience.

Seeking an hEDS diagnosis: Where to start

Ironically, I believe it's because as a community we reach out to one another to share great resources that we can often overwhelm the medical system. Consider the case of Dr. Alissa Zingman, who has EDS herself and treats patients in Maryland. Soon after opening her practice she was overwhelmed by patients once word got out to the patient community seeking help, resulting in a four-year waiting list. The system is overwhelmed and unable to support the needs of the patients.

At the same time, the harsh reality is that many with EDS are simply dismissed by the medical profession. Dr. Alan Spanos spoke for many when he observed, "People with EDS... are sidelined or completely ignored by the medical profession. This is getting worse not better, and will continue to do so. For these conditions, patients themselves have to become the experts, then search for the few educable doctors who will take the time to learn from them, and have enough interest in them to want to help them."

Given the inadequacy of resources available, often-times fellow zebras are our best bet for getting the insight and assistance we need.

Getting a diagnosis is one of the hardest things to accomplish when you suspect you are hypermobile. To help my fellow zebras, I recommend taking the following steps in order to establish whether or not you have hEDS.

CROWDSOURCING EMPOWERS PATIENTS

If you've bounced from doctor to doctor with a difficult-to-diagnose condition or live in a rural area, there are many reasons why you might seek out expert medical advice from a larger community of like-minded people. While patients have long turned to social media to seek answers to their medical questions, there are now more reputable sources than Facebook. Seeking feedback from other patients or getting a second opinion is as easy as going online. While many nonprofits offer hope and information, a few tools are very helpful in bringing the wisdom of many to your fingertips. "Medical crowdsourcing" sites and apps are gaining momentum, including patient-focused sites such as CrowdMed, StuffThatWorks, and PatientsLikeMe. They share the same mission of empowering patients, reducing misdiagnosis, and improving medicine by gathering the greater power of patients' experiences.

Step 1 – Track Your Symptoms

To begin the diagnosis process, you first must pay close attention to your body; notice and document all symptoms no matter how unrelated they might seem to connect the dots and show evidence of patterns and then share with your care team. Write down and journal what ails you, track and log any symptoms, and record things you've tried, whether they worked or failed at treating the issue(s). Documentation is vital to getting a proper diagnosis. I have made available several editable medical templates for varying types of tracking, logging, journaling, appointment preparation, and more for your use that can be found at https://bit.ly/medicaltemplates. Feel free to share.

Step 2 – Use Available Information to Self-Assess

To begin the process of determining whether there is hypermobility, use the suggested resources below to initiate collecting evidence on your own if you think that you might be affected. This information is critical to bring to your medical appointments. Be careful not to become an Internet sleuth and attempt to diagnose yourself—allow the trained medical professional to do that for you, but come armed with data.

- Use this checklist from the EDS Society website to get you started: www.ehlers-danlos.com/heds-diagnostic-checklist;
- Learn about the Beighton scale and score. At present it is the only standard physical evaluation used commonly to test hypermobile joints. The Beighton score

is a simple system to quantify joint laxity and range of motion. It uses a simple 9-point system, where the higher the score, the higher the laxity, with the threshold varying for younger versus older individuals.

- There is a developing tool called "The Spider" according to the Hypermobility Syndromes Association (HMSA), which is a 25-item questionnaire outlining several common symptoms of hypermobility. The result is a graph shaped like a spider web that can help providers see a visual representation of your symptom profile. Although not yet validated as of 2021, evidence is emerging that patients with non-musculoskeletal issues such as fatigue, dysautonomia, and gastrointestinal symptoms have a worse disease progression along the eight areas examined: musculoskeletal, pain, fatigue, gastrointestinal, cardiac dysautonomia, urinary incontinence, depression, and anxiety.

Step 3 – Seek Medical Evaluations, Diagnosis, and Potential Treatment of Symptoms from Medical Specialists

This step can take a long time. The key is preparation. You likely will have only a few precious minutes with the provider to tell your story, share symptoms, and ask questions. Hopefully you won't be dismissed but will instead receive a thorough examination before ordering any testing. That outcome is much more likely if you come prepared with a detailed and thorough accounting of your symptoms.

To adequately prepare for each appointment, follow these guidelines:

- **Read up on your condition**. Knowing typical responses may help you prepare yourself. The more you learn about your illness, the more you'll understand your treatments, emotions, and the best ways to create a healthy lifestyle based on your individual needs.

- **Summarize your issues succinctly**. State clearly up front the goals of your appointment and stay focused on them. Bring in writing a list of your symptoms and a copy of your existing medications (including any supplements you take) organized alphabetically for ease of comparison to your records. Sometimes communicating is hard when you are emotionally invested and feel overwhelmed or have brain fog. I have found it easier to communicate in writing, and it helps me stay focused on the outcomes I want to achieve at each appointment. Be specific in symptom tracking: The nature of symptoms, frequency, location, or type and any effects on your abilities to function are key data points.

- **Ask for an evaluation** if you suspect hypermobile EDS. Bring copies of your interpretation and review of your Beighton scale and diagnostic criterion documents. Remember, you are not at the doctor for validation but for a trained professional to help problem-solve with you.

- **List any concerns** on paper or your phone as a sort of agenda for the appointment. While it is frustrating not being heard by a doctor, it can be equally disorienting to have a doctor really listen to you, and it can throw you off your game with elation! Creating a checklist of the topics you want to cover in the typical 15–20 minute time with the provider is essential for achieving clear and concise communication. Apps are useful and readily available (see my recommendations in Chapter 15).

- **Focus on relief for your worst symptom.** Ask about treatment options, any potential side effects, and interactions with existing medications, allergies, or conditions.

- **Take notes and ask questions**: There's usually a lot of information to absorb when visiting a doctor, and it's overwhelming. I encourage you to take written notes at all major doctor appointments. You want to go over specifics once or ask them to repeat things to be sure you understand everything clearly. This may sound basic, but many people hesitate to say, "Can you say that again?" because they don't want to sound stupid. But it takes doctors years of medical school and practice to learn the information they're passing on to you in a few minutes. For example, you might want to ask how you can expect to respond to prescriptions or treatment because it varies significantly from one person to the next.

- **Bring support**. Given the complex nature of how EDS symptoms present, to a provider we can appear disorganized. Documentation and preparation can help with that, but so does bringing a "member of your tribe" to the appointment to help by taking notes (audio or other recording is not permitted with HIPAA laws without permission) while you concentrate and focus on conversing with the doctor (like many of us, I have a tendency to forget what the doctor said, and notes to look back on have been a lifesaver on more than one occasion). It is also simply a sad fact of life that sometimes the presence of a second individual—especially if that person is a male—changes the tone of an appointment and means you are taken more seriously by providers.

- **Follow up**. Get a copy of your visit or care summary so you can ensure accuracy and recall. Most providers offer online patient portals. Ask for access. If testing is ordered, call your insurance provider to ensure approval in advance to avoid financial surprises. Ask if coverage is for in-network or not. Never disparage a doctor unless you are officially reporting them to your source to stop referrals. Document all activity in your records including medication changes, diagnosis, testing, or referrals to specialists.

Overall, pack a lot of patience as you weed through the medical system through trial and error to find what helps you and your individual EDS symptoms.

THE IMPORTANCE OF HEALTH INSURANCE

I am grateful to have health care insurance currently and a supportive spouse. I understand that we are not all fortunate enough to have good (or even any) health care or family support. As you know, health care in the United States is in a crisis. I have been able to take advantage of health benefits through my previous jobs or have used my husband's insurance to maintain medical coverage. We do pay outrageous amounts for the care we choose, need, and desire and add in extra coverages as we can afford them. We have learned that having accessible medical care benefits is crucial to our quality of life, so we make important life choices to choose employment many times based on insurance options. Do your homework in this very critical area.

Key provider types

Our health care network of specialized siloed practitioners doesn't integrate a single provider to see the whole person or to have a broad perspective. Therefore, it is difficult to diagnose EDS. We go from specialist to specialist for symptoms, and it can take years to get a clue about what's happening to you, how to deal with it, and how to manage the medical system to find treatment. For many people who have fought various dismissive doctors or care providers who exhibited no empathy, this is a truly frustrating experience that can traumatize them. Being repeatedly dismissed as your issues being "all in your head" is overwhelming and can be devastating.

In order to manage many chronic illnesses such as EDS, patients often are forced to tackle the arduous task of seeing a village of different types of specialty providers who focus on different systems within the body. The primary goals in finding the right doctors to treat hEDS are to manage symptoms, prevent joint injury, and educate yourself about your condition. Patients with hypermobile EDS/hypermobility spectrum disorders can benefit from physical and occupational therapy, psychological support, and insight into self-management provided by knowledgeable caregivers.

In my view, the best way to start to get help and start treatment is to determine what are the worst, most unmanageable symptoms and determine what type of specialist to see first by priority of your discomfort. To assist in that effort, below are recommendations on the types of doctors most commonly seen for the symptomatic treatment of the core issue of hypermobility.

These doctors can be found on community forums, by searching online, or by seeking out EDS-related medical provider directories.[1] When you call to book an appointment ask if the provider has a working knowledge of EDS as that understanding is critical to you receiving the care

---

[1] For resources on how to locate provider recommendations, see Chapter 15 on support organizations, which includes a detailed listing of nonprofits that support EDS research and publish provider lists.

you need that supports the complexities zebras face. Keep seeking out a provider until someone really listens to you. You will know when you find the right one.

- **Geneticist:** To be formally diagnosed with EDS, you can see a geneticist. They will run DNA (usually blood or saliva) tests to identify genetic abnormalities found in people with EDS or other connective tissue disorders. This testing can also help to determine someone's EDS subtype. They will conduct a Beighton scale test to determine your level of hypermobility. If you are clearly an hEDS person, then other doctors or even an EDS-experienced physical therapist can use the hEDS diagnostic criteria checklist.

- **Functional medical doctor:** Functional medicine doctors use specialized training and techniques to find the root causes of complex illnesses. They may investigate multiple factors causing a condition, or they may look into multiple conditions causing one symptom. This is helpful to have a holistic review. It's often helpful to have the functional medicine perspective that usually includes testing your blood, hormones, vitamin and mineral deficiencies, and proper functioning of the organs responsible for detoxification of waste in the body. Often, they do not accept insurance, but the perspective they provide can be invaluable. My functional medicine doctor was able to determine I had Epstein-Barr virus and significant estrogen dominant syndrome—and help me fix these issues so I could concentrate on my EDS.

- **Cardiologist:** I highly recommend you find a specialized cardiologist familiar with EDS and its comorbidities of dysautonomia and POTS. There are many tests they can give you to determine whether you have POTS, such as an EKG to monitor your heart rate and blood pressure as well as a tilt table test which is designed to measure the variance of your heart rate between lying down and standing up (warning: it's not fun).

- **Neurologist:** It is essential to see a neurologist to evaluate symptoms causing pinched nerves, joint instability, sleep problems, cognitive declines, or headaches. They can evaluate your sensory systems to determine if you have numbness, tingling, loss of motor control, or balance issues. I could not walk in a straight line, bounced off the walls, had frequent falls, and dropped things for a while—all things my neurologist was able to help me start addressing.

- **Gastroenterologist:** Many people with EDS struggle with gastrointestinal and digestive system issues such as irritable bowel syndrome (IBS). We often have irregular bowel movements, which can wreck our immune system and make us prone to adverse reactions to food, even to an extreme and ultimately get mastocytosis. After allergy dermatology tests and an elimination diet, I learned I had a severe gluten intolerance and was later diagnosed with celiac disease. It took me several years to really get gluten out of everything—not only in the foods I consumed but household products such as toothpaste and cosmetics that touched my skin too. After a couple of years of strict guidance to zero gluten, the daily hives and severe digestive issues ended. (Note: When you see a gastro doctor, remember you still have to be consuming gluten to properly test using endoscopies and/or colonoscopies for gluten intolerance or celiac disease.)

- **Neuro-ophtalmologist:** As we age, we commonly lose our vision a bit, but when you have EDS, your vision and eyes can be significantly affected because your eyes are mostly made of collagen. An ophthalmologist can measure the pressure in the eyes that affects vision and balance. My neuro-ophthalmologist diagnosed me with EDS-related convergence, where my right and left eye could not simultaneously come together to focus on a single object, leading to feelings of nausea whenever I would swivel my head.[2]

- **Physical therapist:** One of the most valuable specialists to see is a physical therapist (PT). I

---

[2] To learn more, read my interview with my EDS-knowledgeable neuro-ophthalmologist, Dr. Eric Singman (former clinical director of the Johns Hopkins Wilmer Eye Institute), in the Healthcare Heroes Summit Appendix.

strongly recommend you find one who understands EDS, as one who doesn't understand the complexities of hypermobility can wind up causing more problems than they solve. Skilled PTs can help teach you new muscle memory and improve your proprioception—the ability to recognize where your body is in space—which is altered in EDS. PTs can also help you learn how to do the exercises at home to manage your pain and frequent subluxations. Being able to care for yourself at home will give you a better sense of control over your own body, which people with EDS often do not feel.[3]

- **Pain management specialist:** Finding the right pain management provider who will give you helpful solutions is paramount to a better quality of life. Be very careful in pain management for obvious reasons of addiction and substance abuse. I share snippets from my interview with the director of the US Pain Foundation in the Appendix, who gives suggestions on coping with chronic pain and creating a pain plan of action to ease flares.

- **Rheumatologist:** A rheumatologist can test for immunity and autoimmunity issues, often diagnoses EDS, and even can refer patients to geneticists if

---

[3] To learn more, read my interview with my hypermobile-specialty trained PT, Dr. Amanda Miller, which you can find in the Healthcare Heroes Summit Appendix.

necessary. They typically evaluate your entire body (including your skin) for abnormalities and conduct antigen-induced arthritis (AIA) tests. (Note: Good rheumatologists understand that autoimmunity and AIA are not always linked.)

- **General practitioner (GP)/primary care physician (PCP):** The most important medical professional on your team is a good GP, PCP, or internist who understands (or is willing to learn about) the idiosyncrasies of EDS and its comorbidities. Primary care physicians play a crucial role not only in initial recognition, diagnosis, and patient education but by virtue of their ongoing relationship, they can also help oversee and coordinate the multidisciplinary team many of these patients require.

My initial recommendation is to find a functional medicine or internist to help you coordinate all of your multisystemic issues. It is very important to have a single doctor, your primary care provider or GP, as the centralized point of contact who collects and reviews your medical history and information overall. This is helpful not only for your care management but for your medical record tracking, which you will need if you plan to file for disability.

I have been fortunate enough to have the same remarkable primary care provider for over 25 years, Dr. Annette Hudler. She strongly recommends that it is critical for anyone with a chronic health condition to document their history and progress. Doing so requires becoming an organized person. You will need to document and write out your medical history, medications, symptoms, family history, and any past surgeries or hospitalizations. You need to keep a calendar of your doctor appointments. She stresses that it is very important to prepare for your doctor appointments so that you make the best use of their time while you have them. Have any questions prepared, any new or changing symptoms prepared in advance to share with your care team, and always bring copies of any recent labs, treatment, reports, or clinical notes with you to each doctor.

The moral of the story is *you* must take responsibility to research and help yourself in the multidisciplinary approach to your care and the variety of your care team members. You are the ringmaster of your own circus. You will find providers who will listen and those who won't. Keep searching and seeking new opinions if you are not satisfied. You have the right to be heard!

> *While we may not be able to choose all the things that happen to us in life, we do get to choose how to react to those things. We get to choose what they mean to us.*
>
> **—Carrie Dale**

Consider hiring a patient advocate

Another option to consider in assisting with your medical care management are patient health advocates. You can find people who work on behalf of specific diseases or former nurses turned advocate who can help navigate the medical system. Their services available for hire are intended to guide you to ease the burden, reduce the red tape, and support you and your loved ones in enhancing your understanding of how the health care system works. I was fortunate enough to access a patient advocate within my health care insurance company that operated on my behalf for free (we all know why—they wanted me to stop being such an expensive claim!). But through the advocate, I received detailed second opinion research into providers who understood EDS, pharmacology guidance, and even help to prepare for medical appointments. Be sure to ask about this resource, especially if you are under the care of a hospital or clinic as it is typically free. Patient advocates can be a lifesaver and can reduce your fear and frustration of medical bills and uncertainty.

I have been so inspired by the EDS community that I am determined to become a patient advocate. I'm pleased to be a part of the Ehlers-Danlos Society's ECHO training on how to advocate for EDS patients as a community leader.

Hear from an advocacy expert

I had the privilege of interviewing the expert and founder of the Alliance of Professional Health Advocates (APHA), Trisha Torrey. If you're looking to find an advocate, her organization has created and manages an online directory of private health care advocates who work on the patient's behalf instead of their allegiance being with the insurance company, hospital, or other party: www.aphadvocates.org/directory. She outlines her best tips in her book *You Bet Your Life: 10 Mistakes Every Patient Makes*.

What guidance do you suggest to patients of any disease or disorder as they navigate the health care system?

- "You need to be a smart patient. The health care world has changed, and nobody's bothered to tell the patients. We go in with a set of assumptions that the system is there to help us. And once we get into it far enough, we realize, no, the system is set up to make money. If they happen to help some patients in the meantime, that's okay too. These are the things you need to do: You need to develop lists of questions for your doctor. You need to do research on your own, but you need to find credible research. Not the stuff that's put out there by the pharmaceutical companies, but the stuff that's put out there that is independent and objective. And you need to be able to read your prescription bottles. And you need to go online and make sure that your prescription doesn't conflict with some other provider's prescription for you, because two doctors don't necessarily look to see what the other one prescribed."

You started your business after you were misdiagnosed with a terminal brain tumor that you later

discovered on your own was a medical error thus avoiding chemo and treatment that would have altered your life. How do you suggest people stand up to the dismissive medical community who sometimes treat us like "it's all in our head?"

- "It's usually females, of almost any age, but it's especially females who have unclear symptoms for which there is not a simple test. It's a lot easier for a doctor who, by the way, is only given ten minutes by your insurance company to talk to you at all. I decided I had to prove it's not in your head. You might say to the doctor, "Okay, if it's in my head, how do we figure out what I can do about that, so it won't be in my head anymore?" They'll refer you to a psychiatrist. Then you go and you have an evaluation with the psychiatrist who then says there's nothing wrong with your head. Then they go back to your original doctor who says, no, it's not in her head. Now the doctor must work with her to get the diagnosis she needs. Sometimes if you face those naysayers head-on by using their tactics, you can often come back around to prove that, in fact, there's a problem here, and you've got to get to the root of it. That's one of the ways you do it. The other way you do it is you work with someone who works specifically with patients who are not getting the information they need, like a patient advocate."

What sorts of things does a patient advocate do for a typical client, whether it's the patient or a caregiver?

- "In a lot of cases, patients are what I call stuck in F.U.D.G.E.—Fear, Uncertainty, Doubt, Guilt, or Exhaustion. Any of those emotions can get in the way of you getting what you need. An awful lot of people are working a full-time job, maybe with kids at home, and also helping an elderly parent. Meanwhile, you've got symptoms that need to be attended to, but you just don't have it in you. At the point where you feel like either you've reached the end of your rope physically or you've reached the end of your rope mentally, or you've reached the end of your resourcefulness. That's the time that you tap into somebody who can fill in those gaps for you. Maybe what you do is you don't just hire them to do all the work for you. Maybe what you do is you hire them to guide you. For example, when you get some sort of bad news, whether that bad news means we can't figure it out or that bad news means a specific diagnosis that will take over just about everything else in your life. So what makes you think you can get the care you need during this difficult time? If you work with someone who can have that clarity of thought, that's really the best approach, I think, to getting exactly what you need out of the system. That's what independent advocates are for."

There are other factors that come into play that people probably don't recognize that advocates bring to light like the allegiance factor. Tell us about that.

- "First of all, we recognize that there are lots of people who can volunteer to help. Those people might be loved ones, they might be neighbors, they might be the nurse who lives down the street or goes to your church or your synagogue. Or they might be a patient advocate who is in hospital. Or it might be the person who's really customer service of the insurance company who says calls themselves a patient advocate, because that's what they're all doing now to make it sound as if somehow, they're going to be able to help you out. Sometimes they are patient advocates who are in pharmaceutical companies. Their sole job is to steer you towards the drugs they've manufactured and sell. There are all these people who don't really work in your best interest. Instead, they work for whoever they work for, who's paying them a paycheck. If you're having a complex procedure, go ask the patient advocate at the hospital. But think again if the patient advocate at the hospital is not serving the needs of the hospital. Trust your gut. Then go find somebody else to help you. If you find that your neighbor who says they can help doesn't really have a good knowledge of the system and how it works, trust your gut. If somebody else has an allegiance somewhere else or doesn't have the know-how to help you out, you're not doing yourself any favors by sticking with them or even trusting them."

In your experience, what might a patient who is chronically ill or an undiagnosed person be able to gain from an advocate as it is a new field? We're accustomed to outsourcing certain tasks, but how do people become interested in engaging an independent patient advocate?

- "That's when I ask them to ponder, 'Okay, if that happened in any other aspect of your life, what would you do?' Suppose you're pulled over on the side of the road by a cop and they haul you off in handcuffs and throw you in jail. And they tell you it's because you were doing X. But you don't really understand that because you don't think you were doing X, but because you argued with them, they've now put you in handcuffs and they've hauled you off to jail. Now what? How do you get out? Next, you're told you have to go to court and you need bail money. Then you must learn how to plead. Who's going to represent you in court? You've been thrown into jail and you've heard about this happening to other people, but you never thought it would happen to you, and you always thought that it wouldn't be anything you would have to deal with. But what do you know instantly? Who is it you should call? A lawyer. Why? Because a lawyer is the person who can navigate you through this system that you've been thrown into that you really don't know anything about. That's the person who's going to represent you when it comes time to fight this. It's not unlike getting thrown into the health care system often the same way when you have symptoms you don't understand, doctors who are speaking a language you don't understand. Who's going to get you out of it? Maybe you'll do it right and maybe you'll do it wrong—you don't know. There are a million pitfalls and a million problems that you're going to run into. If you call an advocate, the advocate is going to help you, and you're going to have to pay the advocate to help you."

Instead of stuffing down your depression, anxiety, shame, loneliness—or whatever emotion you're tempted to resist—ask yourself: What message is it trying to send me? What would I do differently in my life if I listened to this emotion instead of suppressing it.

—Kelly Martin

Self-advocacy: Managing medications and medical records

Today, we have an explosive amount of information at our fingertips. But we must be careful with the power of the

Internet to use it wisely for our health as we advocate and seek answers for ourselves. Here are a few tips regarding self-advocacy and education also from Trisha Torrey:

1. **Follow the money** – In the provider scenario ask yourself who is paying, who to best judge, who can help you best.

2. **Find a second or third confirmation** – There is often unconfirmed information on alternative or other therapies. Do your due diligence before trying anything new.

3. **The HON code** – HON developed a set of legal, ethical, and practical criteria for websites. Make sure any website you use has an HON badge and verify it before following their advice.

4. **Peer-reviewed** – Medical scientists share information in two primary ways—presenting findings at conferences and publishing in medical journals. These journals are typically peer-reviewed, meaning other specialists must attest it is evidence-based. Be very skeptical of therapies that are not peer-reviewed.

5. **Discuss any and all standards of care with your doctors.**

Pharmacology in particular can be a complex area to discuss because most of us are on a variety of different medications to the extent of humiliation. Many EDS sufferers are on muscle relaxers, over-the-counter pain relief, serious pain medication, antidepressants, anti-anxiety, and many other types of drugs. If you also suffer from POTS, then you can add to that prescription list heart medication, beta-blockers, and meds to keep your blood flow optimal. We are often prescribed different medications by various doctors, and no one is looking at the whole picture of what we are taking.

This is a critically important area to become a self-advocate. Have your pharmacist review the full scale and scope of what you're taking and the interactions between them. Have your general practitioner also look over your list regularly and monitor any changes and potential side effects. Also, given that people with EDS tend to metabolize medications at different rates than others, having pharmacogenetic testing done to determine how you metabolize specific drugs can be highly beneficial.

You must rely on your medical care team to manage precisely which prescriptions are best for your individual case to take and at what dosages. But you have to be your own advocate to make sure your medication is meeting your needs. Medication is a necessary evil of chronic illness. The EDS population is likely to be on some form of multiple medications for life. That is a tough pill to swallow emotionally. At the same time, one of the most essential things for someone with EDS is to actually take your medication! This means you have to have the cognitive ability to be able to keep up with it, which can be a daunting task and create feelings of shame. This is an area where it is really hard to ask for help.

One of the ways that I overcame past challenges in managing my medications was to get a large enough weekly pill case. This was emotionally hard to do. I suggest you don't judge yourself and just break down and do it. You may find it helpful to install a prescription management reminder tool or app on your phone such as Medisafe so you can enter all of your prescriptions, times taken, and dosage. These can help you track when you take medications with helpful pop-up reminders. Many also have features that monitor when you miss doses historically and even let you share your data with your doctor.

It is important to follow your doctor's orders and take advantage of all the tools they provide to help you. But keep in mind it is possible to get off medications. I'm thrilled to report that I'm off 85 percent of my previous prescribed medications and supplements through following my healthy habits.

The most important thing to finding the root cause of your disease is understanding and documenting your symptoms and working with your care team to look for patterns. You must make the serious investment of time to know, understand, and create your entire medical profile. This critical ongoing task, which can be daunting, boils down to one of my best recommendations: **You must maintain your own detailed medical records.**

Managing your medical care is both your legal right and ultimately your responsibility. Ask for copies of everything from your medical providers: all your lab, testing, and imagining results, as well as doctors' clinical and any progress notes from your visits. Scan and digitize it, organize it, back it up to the cloud and occasionally review it to recognize long-term patterns as well as any potential errors in the doctors' notes. I also recommend that you keep a living document of all the medications you're taking with notes on why and how often you're taking it, who prescribed it, and when you started taking it. This is an excellent tool at doctor appointments to review your meds and can be helpful if you ever have to go to the hospital (it also could be potentially life-saving if your emergency contact had a copy of your medications).

Creating and managing such documents is a huge task and a pain, and this is just another example of why having a chronic illness sometimes feels like an exhausting full-time job. But your records will prove to be invaluable when your memory fails you.

Choose to Assess, Act, or Affirm

- **Assess:** What good benefits do you receive from any of the medications you are currently taking? How might they have changed your life for the better?

- **Act:** Try downloading the app MyLinks to create a digital record file of your personal medical records. It is sharable temporarily with people you designate and secure by HIPAA regulations.

- **Affirm:** "The treatments I follow are helping my body to heal."

Bibliography

Torrey, T. (2013). *You Bet Your Life!: The 10 Mistakes Every Patient Makes*. DiagKNOWsis Media.

NOTES

CHAPTER 6

MIRACLES OF THE MODERN MINDSET

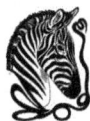

---

*Kristin Neff defines self-compassion as "being warm
and understanding toward ourselves when we suffer,
fail, or feel inadequate, rather than ignoring our
pain or flagellating ourselves with self-criticism."
No positive change can happen in an atmosphere
of criticism and self-abuse. We can't force ourselves
to do better. We have to offer ourselves support and
encouragement to heal and grow.*

—Joanna Ciolex

While we can look at research that shows some potential
benefits of a positive mindset and linkages between
the level of a person's optimism and things like their
health and longevity, it doesn't take a rocket scientist to

tell us what we already inherently know. We know that if we think more positively and feel more optimistic, everything else in our life feels a little bit (or a lot) easier.

I am advocating for "cautious optimism" in your wellness journey. There is a delicate balance between optimism and realism. I recognize that thinking positively will not necessarily get you out of the requirement for your mobility aids, for example, but your approach to chronic illness can help you cope with the fact you need one better.

This is not ableism or toxic positivity. I profess to seek out the silver linings among the clouds. Be real and honest with yourself, but try to find the good things in your altered life plan. For example, maybe you met different people in your life as a result of becoming chronically ill?

Maybe you have support you didn't expect? Maybe you learned to appreciate the grace of what you do have instead of what you don't? Find your reason, and give yourself hope.

But if we can improve our reality by enhancing our state of mind, why don't we all just do it? Personally, when I've been told to just think positively and all will be better, my usual reaction is to roll my eyes and say that thinking positively will not cure a genetic mutation or pop a subluxed rib back into place. I fully appreciate how you feel, and it happens to me too. I understand how our bodies cannot do what we want and how simple tasks such as cleaning our homes have become unmanageable and too painful.

But I propose that we all have a better chance of coping more successfully if we believe in the art of the possible. I never got anywhere complaining. In fact, I lost a lot. No success came from that. It is the process of becoming more abundant in our thinking by creating your own world where you can see the silver linings in even the darkest clouds. I understand when you are in a great deal of pain this sounds insurmountable. But you can train your brain.

There are two things you need to know about retraining your brain. The first is that no one is born an optimist, and no one is born a pessimist. These are **learned** ways of being and behaving, which we pick up throughout life based on how our mindset was conditioned. As a consciously aware adult, you get to **choose** and recondition your mind to whatever outlook you prefer. I had to relearn this programming myself.

The second thing to know is that optimism is **not** denying reality. It's not being caught up in la-la land filled with rainbows, fairies, and unicorns. It is a deliberate choice to keep one's mind and heart open to bring conscious awareness, free will, and the possibility to any situation we may face. It is the intelligence to know that our perception influences our life outcomes and that we alone are responsible for our empowerment. It is taking the realistic view.

Don't get me wrong; I am not suggesting that optimism will cure what ails you. But in the spirit of the art of the possible, I do believe that even small changes can make a big difference in your life. Those small changes have helped me a lot, including giving me a new outlook on life and living with chronic illness. This is what led

THE FALLACY OF MEASURING YOUR PRODUCTIVITY

I have lived most of my adult life driven by a to-do list, buying various sizes and shapes of planners and lists to better organize my thoughts and tasks. It wasn't until I learned to stop living this way that I really started to change.

There is an excellent article from the online resource Tiny Buddha where the blog author, Nancy Daley, writes that she struggled with the same.

> Most of us will measure our day by what we did. We will reflect back and count the things on the to-do list we could check off. The more checkmarks, the better. How well we did will also come into play as we reflect back on our doing. The more praise we received for it, either the self-provided kind or that offered by others, the higher we rank our day in terms of quality.

If you struggle from this sense of self-worth being mandated by what you accomplished, and even worse, when you can no longer achieve those things due to chronic illness, cut yourself a break.

me to write a survival guide that gives individuals with EDS a sense of hope in the possibilities of the future. Better yet is the fact that being optimistic is entirely free and requires no equipment, technology, appointments, co-pays, prescriptions, or anything. Why not try working on changing your mindset? What do you have to lose?

The fine art of learning from obstacles

Life is full of obstacles. Chronic illness can be a considerable one.

For most people, obstacles are one of the more challenging aspects of life. We set goals with enthusiasm and energetically take action to achieve them. Everything looks great for a while. Then it happens: the setback. The hurdle in the way. We've been stalled out and suddenly have no idea what to do next. Things come grinding to a halt, and the world feels like it's coming to an end. A diagnosis of an incurable chronic illness can lead to thoughts like that.

When you hear the word "obstacle," an obstacle course might come to mind. As a child, you probably played on several such courses. You might have even created your own with branches and rocks, setting up various challenges in your backyard or on the playground. When a child is confronted with an obstacle course, they never pause to consider the possibility of stopping. They charge full speed ahead, and when they come to something blocking their progress to the finish line, they look at it as a challenge, a puzzle, something to get through, or up, or over until they are on the other side. Every obstacle becomes an opportunity to show off their physical prowess and thinking skills to their friends. It's a way of saying, "Watch me do this!"

In the adult world, though, obstacles aren't always so clear-cut. They take on many forms and seem to be absolutely everywhere. At some point, we get burned out from trying, overwhelmed with the sheer work involved in getting through, and eager to take the excuse to just walk away. Obstacles look like too much work, and regardless of the payoff, we're just no longer interested in pushing through. What is it about growing up that teaches us obstacles can stop our dreams in their tracks?

Most of our challenges come when we feel like we don't have enough resources or time to do the things we want to do and need to do. Frustration builds, especially when we get stuck in a cycle of trying to please everyone all the time, forgetting our own goals are just as legitimate and necessary as anyone else's.

When participants in a study were asked to list the challenges they faced regularly, they came up with items that included:

- Tension at work;
- Worries about health;
- Not getting it right;
- Not enough hours in the day;

- Problems with boss/co-workers;
- Lack of funds to cover basic needs;
- Demands from children;
- Being overcommitted;
- Lack of energy;
- Needing to be in two places at once.

Sound familiar? Chances are you can probably come up with an additional item or two that is bothering you right now. And truth be told, doing the hard work to heal from a chronic illness and recover your life is easily avoided and can become an obstacle. Who wants to focus on illness?

But sometimes (if you allow it and in fact encourage it to happen), obstacles become not so much a stopping point as a new challenge—an opportunity to discover something new about yourself or about the world you live in. Obstacles are what creates growth and make life more enjoyable as the hero struggles to reach the peak of their existence.

It's a radical thought, isn't it?

Many of life's obstacles are decidedly out of our control, but some of them are things we can do something about. We can learn the art of turning obstacles into opportunities. Obstacles are what help us to grow. If life were always easy, we'd never reach our best selves. Obstacles make us stronger, teach us lessons, and make us more persistent.

When we meet with an obstacle, our reaction tells the world about who we really are. It's here where we're seen at either our best or our worst. Are you courageous? Do you have a steel backbone? Do you hide when confronted with trouble? Do you run away? These are the (sometimes brutal) truths about us we can only learn when we're put to the test. Here we either prove ourselves or understand where we need work. **Had we never been challenged, we never would have had the opportunity to know who we really are.**

Once we have learned these truths about ourselves, we know what needs work. Obstacles are what are going to give you the skills to create a better version of yourself. Nothing teaches patience like an opportunity to be patient. Nothing will instruct you in bravery better than the moment you stand up to what scares you. These are the crucial pieces of who we are inside. Without the obstacle, we never would have had the opportunity to learn these truths about ourselves.

Sometimes what's blocking us comes from within. What makes these hurdles particularly interesting is the fact that we might have some measure of control over them. This doesn't mean winning out over health challenges is necessarily going to be easy or even doable, though. We indeed are our own worst enemies, and frequently these challenges come with a lot of baggage and even more work to deal with them. But aren't you worth a try?

Obstacles teach us persistence. We learn very little when things go along smoothly. If the first effort yields the result we want right away, there's never any cause to try again. We start thinking everything should involve immediate gratification and that nothing should take personal effort. Obstacles teach us how to try again. And then they teach us how to try after that, and after that. When we have to expend the effort to get past the blockage, we learn how to become diligent in our efforts. We know nothing comes without a cost, nor should everything just be given to us. We understand the value of hard work. Obstacles teach us the importance of an exceptional work ethic and how to keep going when the going gets tough.

The occasional obstacle has a way of really forcing us to adjust. These obstacles teach us how to be more creative in our approach. By being forced to think outside the box, we exercise portions of our brain that might not be used as often as we'd like. We become more inclined to have brilliant ideas and put things together in ways we wouldn't usually. We consider new alternatives and explore options we might never have gone down before.

While these various challenges might seem impossible, they frequently aren't. If you're willing to put in the work, there are solutions for almost every problem. For example, the financial burden of medical costs may seem insurmountable. But what if you adjusted your spending, found a new or higher-paying job, filed for disability support, or even considered bankruptcy protection. Have you investigated resources to assist such as NeedyMeds, or applying for scholarships from charitable organizations? It may sound simplistic with complicated and life-altering health problems, escalating medical bills, lack of health insurance, and so many of our expectations out of whack. But in truth there are many ways to try to ease the burden—too numerous to list (though many are listed in Chapter 15 about support). None of them are easy and all require work—and a mindset attuned to possibilities.

I'm not going to lie or sugarcoat it—this is back-breaking work. But who is more worth it than you? Try to be open-minded as you read, think outside of your box of pain, and believe life can be worth living again.

When we have to fight for what we have, and every accomplishment is an arduous journey taking profound effort, we come to really appreciate what we have when it's all over. We learn the gratitude that comes from pushing the envelope. The lessons don't stop there, though. We start to appreciate the efforts of those around us. We understand their struggles better and have more compassion for what they're going through. We're more grateful when they choose to make us part of their journey and appreciate the gifts they have to share with us. Gratitude makes us better people in a soul-edifying way we would never know had the obstacle not allowed us to learn.

My most important advice is to never give up. Don't stick your head in the sand and hope your illness goes away. Fight and find answers, try recommended treatments to see what works for you. See other specialists until someone helps you (as long as you can get to the appointment and have resources to pay the out-of-pocket costs or co-pays/deductibles). Connect with research hospitals doing clinical research and patient trials on your diagnosis to get free or discounted care. Ask for help when you need it from the community of other patients. Locate financial resources from places such as the Patient Advocate Foundation.

It's obstacles such as health issues that can flatten us. When the world is spiraling out of control, and we feel like we can no longer stand up under the winds buffeting us, we eventually have to learn how to let go. When we have accomplished these things, this is the moment we have attained inner peace. Obstacles are an opportunity to embrace humility and to let go of things we have no control over, freeing us to focus on the things we can change. **This is where the key to healing begins, and tenacity is key. Be resilient. And be kind to yourself, but learn to let some of the small stuff go. Focus on you and your health.**

This guide can help you get through those rough places, including your battle with chronic illness diagnoses, and their challenges. We will cycle through a lot of detail on things you can do to better your life with chronic illness. You can learn how to take on the obstacles in your life and turn them into opportunities.

BECOMING A PATIENT PATIENT

I'm working on having more patience. I tend to want everything to be done immediately and perfectly, which—as you can imagine—doesn't go over well. It is ingrained in our instant gratification lifestyle and has led me to a life of unmet expectations, disappointments, and frustration. It's challenging when you are on long waiting lists to see specialist doctors waiting for tests and helpful treatment. For me, it's been the hardest lesson to learn.

A fundamental mindset shift required to better cope with chronic illness is learning to become "a patient patient." I believe it is a critical skill to develop to thrive and survive. Learning to take it day by day, hour by hour, or even minute by minute is a key insight for those with chronic illness to learn. Learn to be patient with the medical system, doctors, waiting for test results, long waiting times to see specialists, and with yourself. If you gain nothing else from the book—my best advice I can share is to become a patient patient. I do not mean to stop advocating for yourself. I mean for you to allow the unfortunate time it takes to get through grief, waiting lists, and treatment trials and tribulations. I suggest you repeat this in your head every time you sit alone in a doctor's office for long periods. "I am a patient patient." Repeat it thousands of times in your head.

The healing habits

In the words of Charles Darwin, "It is not the strongest of the species that survives [...] It is the one that is most adaptable to change." Accepting obstacles is a means to change.

My health and wellness are not separate from the rest of my day. I have a daily and weekly routine and habits I have formed on purpose, and my health and wellness play an integral part. I balance my daily routine by taking everything that needs to happen on that day—work, relationships, home, parenting, living, and my health. Everything can change when you start living with your own well-being in mind. Habits become our routines and behaviors and can form a rhythm of slow methodical change that is doable.

I healed my life by changing my basic daily routines— routines that I refer to as my Ms. Not the candy-coated chocolate candies, although I did enjoy a few peanut M&Ms® along the way. The strategies of my M's that I use have simply helped me to live a better life, a more fulfilling one, with less pain, injury, struggle, and disappointment. I changed my thinking and retrained my brain away from pain. What we desire can manifest itself when we tie our minds to our body's goals.

The Ms started as the easiest way in the beginning for me to remember what I needed to focus on. A simple mnemonic tool. I could keep my brain fog focused on which of the Ms I would do that day. I have significant cognitive issues, especially remembering things, so I would repeat these Ms in my head each day, multiple times a day, to focus on moving, meditating, meals, etc. They naturally formed an "M" repeating mantra for me. Some days, sometimes for months, it is all I could do to remember a few of the Ms. I had to post them on my fridge to remind me of the most important things for me to focus on.

This led to the development of what I call lovingly the **Meltdown Method (MM).** I call it the Meltdown Method for two reasons. First, I basically had to have a meltdown in my own life to reach the lowest level possible to realize what I needed to do to recover. It then took melting down all the facets of my life to learn how to strip away the excess and focus on the bare bones of what I needed to do simplistically that would get and keep me healthy.

The Meltdown Method is a set of habits you can use to rebuild your wellness. If you treat the potential renewal with the same tenacity you might give a new program in self-help and development or how you approach doctors, you can achieve similar results.

Much like the tastiest dishes in the kitchen laden with fat and sugar to taste better, life itself has a lot of excess. You can define your own areas of excess and choose to trim the fat. Mine included harmful ingredients I chose to cut out like toxic relationships, social media, comparing myself to healthy capable friends, and unmanageable stress. I discovered that melting away the layers led me to core principles of what I needed to get better. That meant focusing on just a few simple things: rest, healthy food, exercise as I can tolerate it, and a healthy mindset. Forrest

Gump taught us that life is like a box of chocolates, you never know what you're gonna get. Make the ones you choose worth the effort.

You can meltdown to the basic core elements of what you deserve and need. And let the rest melt away.

I began with the arduous work of changing my daily behaviors. No magic pills or treatments but lifestyle changes. I changed my habits. Success is the sum of habits. I am not cured, and never will most of us be. But we can choose to get back to baseline or get back to a state of "good."

You *can* create your own new, better life through simple daily habits that make significant changes in your well-being over time. I want you to look into your everyday life and really honestly evaluate your self-care and well-being. What are you eating? Are you drinking enough water? Are you moving at least a little bit every day?

In James Clear's *Atomic Habits: An Easy & Proven Way to Build Good Habits & Break Bad Ones*, he shares his perspective on growing one percent better every day. His book outlines a framework to self-improvement on any goal—health, wealth, etc.—by applying practical strategies to changing your routines. He believes that tiny changes lead to remarkable results by compounding the effects of these small habit changes. That is the type of change I recommend a chronically ill patient take on. Small, steady, well-paced changes that improve your life for the better. As Mary Gutierrez observes, "Small things add up. Small

THE POWER OF POSITIVE AFFIRMATIONS

Positive affirmations are not nonsense—they are scientifically proven to help. The trick is finding affirmations that you can believe in, which actually work when you're confronting a chronic illness. You can do this because your brain is neuroplastic. In basic terms, this means that your brain can rewire its neural pathways and form new connections for the better (or for the worse). An effective way to help your brain become stronger, more resilient, and geared for success is with the information you feed it. That is why affirmations can be a powerful tool if you use them properly. I believe affirmations should be:

- Believable and realistic;
- Practical enough to repeat in your head;
- Easy enough to remember in concept;
- Specifically focused on your journey and;
- Comforting to hear and soothing.

Five chronic illness affirmations to try repeating to yourself...

- I have the mind, heart, and soul of a warrior.
- I look forward to each new day as it gives me a unique chance to grow.

- I am creative, strategic, and resilient – all qualities needed to manage a chronic illness.

- I know that when I want to quit, I won't. When you're ready to quit, it's usually the moment right before miracles happen.

- I know the word "disease" can be broken down to "dis" and "ease." Therefore, I make decisions to help me be in a state of ease in life. I ask my body, "Where are you at ease now?" instead of focusing on where I'm in pain.

things make bigger things. Small things create ripples. Start where you are with what you have."

I also want you to pinpoint certain habits you feel are harmful. You know the ones I'm talking about—the inner critic, the couch potato, the incessant worrier—those that don't contribute to your health goals. If your negative habits didn't come to mind immediately, it could mean you're not quite ready to let go of stuff that brings you pleasure, and that can be sabotaging. **Below you can see the results I achieved by doing so, but read Parts III–V only when you are ready to change.**

My results

Below is a summary of the results I achieved due to working regular healing habits (described in the rest of the book) into my routines.

- I am no longer dizzy sitting still.
- I no longer lose my balance, wobble, or fall down for no reason.
- I no longer require regular hourly horizontal rest periods.
- I no longer get pre-syncope or pass out.
- I no longer have nausea for no reason.
- I no longer require an immobilizing neck brace.
- I no longer have to ice/heat every single day to reduce inflammation.
- I no longer have severe pain in my neck and shoulders.
- I no longer struggle with vision loss including convergence.
- I no longer have tachycardia, and my heart rate went from 150 BPM to the mid-50s.
- I no longer take medications such as antidepressants, anxiety meds, beta-blockers, muscle relaxers, and most pain medication.
- I got my appetite back and gained weight.
- I can gently and carefully exercise every day.
- I can climb the stairs again.
- I can drive my car again for short periods.
- I sleep much better and awake restored.

- I have recovered from major depression and frequent anxiety.

- I have improved cognitively.

- I prioritize self-care.

- I feel an enhanced sense of well-being.

I know I'm not the typical case, and everyone has their own unique issues they face with hypermobility. But through the habits below I made genuine strides and think you can too.

How did I do it? Habits are the culmination of activities we do consistently. To heal myself, I started very small with micro-habits. First, I started drinking more water (now I'm up to over a gallon a day, which with added salt has really helped my blood flow). I noticed I felt better in time, so I added something else. I started moving my body in ways that I could for even just a few minutes per day. In about ten days or so, I noticed that it was having the positive effects of helping me feel better and improving my mood and disposition.

I kept adding more habits the next month—simple yet effective habits such as eating the proper diet and not focusing on the difficulties I was facing—and that turned my thinking around and helped my body heal. I also practiced habit stacking to make it more manageable. It's the art of combining your current habits with new ones you want to start. Take something you already do every day, and pair it with a simple new one you want start doing every day. For example, you may already make coffee every morning, and you also want to work out more—link the two in order to create a routine of your daily habits.

I added some more habits the following month, and so on, and just like that, my sense of well-being soared by comparison. It did take a while, but over the course of a year I truly started to change. I added new habits as I could, and eventually my Ms were formed.

Change is hard. I know. But I also know the last year writing this book has been one of the most remarkable of my entire life. Just one year ago, I was chasing a craniocervical instability diagnosis I didn't know I needed. I only knew I was falling, always nauseous, losing my abilities, and in a great deal of pain. Now I am able to stand before you confessing my fears and imparting a few pieces of wisdom from my own healing Ms that helped me find peace, persistence, and passion. Stay focused on living a joyful life each day and live it one day at a time. Remember, the journey is up to you. Navigate your inner GPS. You've got this.

Choose to Assess, Act, or Affirm

- **Assess:** Are you ready to look at life in a new way?
- **Act:** What can you do now to become an agent of change for yourself?
- **Affirm:** Challenge your beliefs. For example...

  Old Conditioned Belief: "I'm not good enough."
  New Counter-Attack Affirmations: "People love me, and I know that I am enough."

Old Conditioned Belief: "I'm always sick."

New Counter-Attack Affirmations: "I am happy, healthy, and whole. My body is strong, and I am safe within it."

Old Conditioned Belief: "I'm afraid, and I am weak."

New Counter-Attack Affirmations: "I am free of worry, and I grow stronger and more relaxed each day."

Old Conditioned Belief: "Life is hard."

New Counter-Attack Affirmations: "I approach life with ease and grace and am open to learning new lessons along the way. I give thanks for the blessings I receive each day."

Bibliography

Daley, Nancy, and Denney, A. "Measuring the Quality of Your Day with a To-Be List (Not Just a To-Do List)." Tiny Buddha. https://tinybuddha.com/blog/measuring-the-quality-of-your-day-with-a-to-be-list-not-just-a-to-do-list/.

"Chronic Illness: Sources of Stress, How to Cope." https://my.clevelandclinic.org/health/articles/4062-chronic-illness.

Clear, J. *Atomic Habits: An Easy & Proven Way to Build Good Habits & Break Bad Ones*. Penguin Publishing Group, 2018.

NOTES

PART III

LEARNING TO HEAL

In this part, I look closely at the phenomenon of stress: not so much its causes (we know *why* we're stressed) but *how and what* it can do to a hypermobile person and what you can do to prevent it and address it when it strikes. We must understand the ways in which chronic stress—the twenty-first century's black plague—has become one of the leading causes of death, leading to strokes and heart attacks along with a variety of other suboptimal outcomes, from decreased immunity to insomnia, anxiety, depression, addiction, obesity, heart disease, and serious illness. But there's good news too. We can also discover the ways in which certain animals such as zebras have adapted to living marvelously well under pressure!

In these next three chapters I will widen your understanding of how stress and our survival mechanisms interplay. There are suggestions on how to calm and reset your autonomic nervous system, including the dysregulation in POTS, including insights into stress reduction methods such as mindful meditation to reconstruct your healing.

CHAPTER 7

MASTERING STRESS

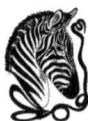

Sit down and write down all the things you're worried/stressed about. Then pretend like you're coaching someone else with those problems. What advice would you give them? What steps would you have them take? Then, follow this step and stop there. Don't worry about whether or not you did enough. You followed your own advice, and you can relax about the rest.

—Kari Dhalgren

I strongly believe stress management is one of the most essential things to regain your health and wellness over-all. The American Psychological Association says when considering the physical and emotional toll of increased stress, nearly half of adults (49%) report their behavior has been negatively affected. Respondents noted increased tension in their bodies (21%), "snapping" or getting angry very quickly (20%), unexpected mood swings (20%), and screaming or yelling at a loved one (17%).

Stress and survival

The priority of any living thing is survival, and the filter most information confronts first is our amygdala – our threat detector. To keep us safe, the amygdala is strongly biased toward negative information. As humans, we're always hunting danger. In experiments run at the University of California, Berkeley, psychologists discovered that we take in as many as nine instances of negative information for every positive one that gets through. Nine-to-one are crappy odds under the best of conditions, and our peak performance rarely takes place under the best of conditions. Yet negative thinking leads to heightened stress. This can crush optimism and squelch your creativity. When turned toward the negative, we miss the fun of experiencing novelty—the foundation for pattern recognition and, by extension, the basis of creativity and solutions.

Before I truly felt the ravages of EDS, stress to me was simply being busy. I worked decades in corporate environments where people use stress as a badge of honor. People proudly commented how busy they were, how many emails were waiting in their inbox, or how many meetings they had. It was like an annoyance always there picking away at you. I thought you just pushed through.

In my case stress built up into so much physical pain it began to interfere with my life. It destroyed my ability to enjoy or continue to attend family events, such as going to the movies or visiting my brother or parents. It killed my entire social circle of friends as I couldn't do fun things anymore. As a driven and ambitious woman who

ALLOSTATIC OVERLOAD

Allostatic load refers to the cumulative burden of chronic stress and life events can have on someone over time. The effects of stress are cumulative and over time these physiological adaptations cause significant wear-and-tear on your body that can negatively affect your immune system, metabolic processes, and cardiovascular system. Allostatic processes lead to increases in blood pressure, lipids, glucose, and inflammation, all of which lead to increased overall health risks, disease, or death.

In *Psychology Today*, Dr. Shawn M. Burn says our physiological stress response helps us respond and adapt to stress. "In fact, it's remarkable how much stress we can bear. But it's not without consequence," he remarks. In other words, your body pays for the lifetime of stress. It's estimated that stress plays a role in anywhere from 50 to 70 percent of all physical illnesses.

self-proclaimed to be very busy, I had to make the choice to set new and different goals to reduce stress in my life post diagnosis. You will likely also need to realign your personal goals and learn new coping skills to overcome chronic illness.

Suggested simple stress management tips

Below are ten stress management tips from licensed clinical social worker and wellness expert Sharon Martin that may be helpful to you in living with chronic illness. Each aim to help you follow the old adage of "saving your spoons for the most important things." Use those that work best for you and alter them as you need to meet your needs.

1. **Learn to let some things go.** When you're going through an intense period of stress, such as working on getting a diagnosis, some things are simply not going to get done. Allow yourself to recognize that you don't have the time or the energy to keep up with everything. If possible, hire help, ask friends to pitch in, and use technology to automate as many things as you can. Come to accept that there will always be things that you can't keep up with.

2. **Don't ridicule yourself.** It's not ideal if your dishes are dirty or the laundry piles up, but sometimes your energy needs to be elsewhere.

3. **Simplify your life.** Because your resources are already stretched thin, be selective about what you

spend your time and energy on. It helps to keep things such as your schedule as simple, routine, and decision-free strategy as possible. Establishing your boundaries is very important as you adjust your life to chronic illness. Focus on doing only what's absolutely essential and grow comfortable declining social invitations, family gatherings, weddings, and learn to say no to additional responsibilities. The rest will have to wait, or someone else will have to do it.

4. **Minimize making any critical decisions.** Making decisions takes a great deal of mental energy, and the more decisions you make, the more energy you expend. Think in terms of having reserves. To the extent possible, try to minimize decisions by keeping things simple. Postpone making big decisions until you're calmer, well-rested, and centered.

5. **Try not to get too hungry, thirsty, or tired.** When your basic needs are met, everything else runs better. Take care of these basic needs first and foremost. We all get grumpy and unfocused quickly when we're hungry, thirsty, and tired. Keep a supply of healthy snacks and water (and electrolytes) in your bag, desk, and car, so you always have them handy. Try to have a consistent sleep schedule and wake at the same time every day, even on weekends—and if you need a nap, take one!

6. **Inform people that you won't be responding as quickly (or at all).** The response time expectations of

today's digital world are ridiculous, both personally and professionally. Don't feel obligated to return every text or email that you get. Silence or mute your phone and put a message on your voicemail and an autoresponder on your email, letting people know that you won't be responding for a while. Then you have the time and the choice to respond when you feel up to it and when it's convenient for you rather than on someone else's time line. This can help with feelings of being overwhelmed and is one way to feel more in control and minimize distractions.

7. **Ask for and accept help.** Accepting help is hard for a lot of people. Asking for help isn't weak; it's a powerful and wise thing to do when you're not at your best. Agreeing to let your friend pick up your kids from school or sit with you during a medical procedure isn't going to solve all your problems, but it can make a significant impact. It may take others a while to understand the types of help you might need, but you can teach them. Being vulnerable when asking for help can help strengthen our serenity and our relationships. Many times it helps others better understand us and our feelings. Remind yourself that people want and like to help too. Allow them the opportunity to be supportive.

8. **Avoid temporary fixes and coping strategies that feel good now but add stress in the long**

run. We all know that overeating, smoking, drinking, and excessive amounts of caffeine aren't healthy ways to cope with stress. It's natural to occasionally seek comfort in these ways, but beating ourselves up later for unhealthy coping strategies will only add more pressure. Be mindful and honest with yourself about how much you're relying on methods that feel good at the moment but cause you more problems in the long haul.

9. **Get it out of your head and on paper to forget about it.** When we're under stress, our short-term memory can suffer. Although this is highly frustrating, it is normal to not recall your doctor's instructions for a new medication or when your next appointment is. Do yourself a favor and write everything down, from the important to the routine. Keep a pad of paper in your purse or on your person, use a note-taking app on your phone, record voice memos, email reminders to yourself, and even take photos of basic things such as where you parked the car.

10. **Seek help.** You can find help for stress-related chronic illnesses. Counseling options include support groups, individual counseling, and/or family and couples counseling. Each can provide an environment where you can learn new ways of dealing with your illness from other people's successful coping strategies. You'll know that you aren't facing hardships alone.

I suggest searching for EDS support groups by contacting a nonprofit organization like those listed in Chapter 15. **Note**: Keep in mind sometimes a support group turns into a collection of naysayers who can suck you into seeing the whole picture negatively and cause you to lose hope. Chronic illness is a bitch, but don't let it turn you into one.

There are some excellent proactive coping skills suggestions in Faith G. Harper's book *Coping Skills: Tools & Techniques for Every Stressful Situation*. She humorously teaches stress self-soothing tools that disarm our defense mechanisms.

When I was diagnosed with EDS, I had to learn new methods to release stress. I examined every habit I had formed that wasn't pushing me to my daily goals and consciously replaced them with activities and exercises that I could obsessively turn into good healing habits.

For example, in the past, a big part of my life was exercising regularly. I have always enjoyed it and used it to release tension at the end of a busy day. I would hold tight muscles in nearly every part of my body, even when sleeping. I didn't know then that my muscles were constantly contracting to hold my joints in place because they were unstable. My parents were always telling me to "loosen up." And so to stretch my muscles, I would exercise, and continue to this day to help me release stress.

Don't get me wrong—I was never fit or even capable of running if a rabid dog was chasing me, but I like the rhythm of exercising and the state it puts me into with the pace of walking, biking, swimming, or yoga. My favorite part then and now is the stretching after. Maybe my body knew it needed extra bending and shaping to heal even back then.

Put yourself at the top of your to-do list every single day, and the rest will fall into place.

—Unknown

The importance of gratitude

Reducing stress is critical, but it's only the first step. Shifting your focus away from stress toward something else can help tremendously as well. How can we teach ourselves better stress management and coping skills? It starts with you and your self-talk in your mind. Oprah has been shouting the benefits of gratitude from the rooftops for decades, and she is right. Positive self-talk with an optimistic outlook on life is one potential solution to chronic stress.

Gratitude is a potent brain trick. A daily gratitude practice can actually alter the brain's negativity bias. It changes the amygdala's filter, essentially training it to take in more positive and refocus the aperture of information coming in. This works very well because the positive stuff you're grateful for is stuff that has already happened in your life and therefore your bullshit detector never gets tripped.

Being grateful enables us to savor positive experiences, cope with difficult circumstances, have higher resilience to stress, and strengthen social

relationships. **The greater the number of gratitude experiences people have on a given day, the better they feel overall, with a deeper feeling of satisfaction with life.**

Research shows that those who practice gratitude—whether through reflection, writing, or in everyday life—report higher levels of positive emotions and a stronger sense of connection. What's even more surprising is that they also have more robust immune systems, lower blood pressure, and experience fewer feelings of loneliness. When we foster a sense of gratitude and appreciation, we inhabit the present moment more fully. This is the unique shift of actually feeling the emotion of appreciation. When we feel grateful, it's challenging to have an opposite emotion. Try being anxious and thankful at the same time—it just doesn't work!

Anna Hennings, a mental performance coach in sports psychology, recommends using the acronym GIFTS to help you identify what you're grateful for. When thinking about things you're grateful for, look for instances of:

- Growth: personal growth, such as learning a new skill;
- Inspiration: moments or something that inspired you;
- Friends/family: people who enrich your life;
- Tranquility: the small, in-between moments, such as enjoying a cup of coffee or a good book;
- Surprise: the unexpected or a nice favor.

There are many ways to start a gratitude practice—here are two that have worked for me:

> **Option one:** Write down ten things you're grateful for quickly, and each time you write an item down, take the time to really feel that appreciation. Try to feel the emotion in your body, discovering where it lives in the body (your gut, your head, your heart) and exactly how it presents itself. Enjoy the moment by recalling a pleasant memory.

> **Option two:** Jot down three things you're grateful for and expand one into a descriptive paragraph or talk about it with another person. I call this "my top 3 of the day," and we share ours as a family at our dinner table nearly every night. It promotes positivity. Focus as before on the somatic nature of your gratitude and where you feel it.

Both approaches will start to shift your perception of the world a bit in small and very gratifying ways, tilting the positivity ratio in a more optimal direction. And it doesn't take long. The research shows that as little as three weeks of daily gratitude is enough to start the rewiring in your brain.

Like many things in life, apps can make tracking gratitude easier. I use an app called Three Good Things, which is very simplistic and low-tech. It allows me to capture every morning the top three things I am most grateful for from the previous day's reflection. Gratitude Journal is a great app that gives you prompts to list what you are thankful for. You can keep your entries private or share them on social media. Gratitude Journal 365 is an app where you can add a daily photo to your entry and view them later for a beautiful display of the things you appreciate.

But while gratitude has several benefits, it can also bring a sense of guilt if we don't feel grateful. Here are some common pitfalls to avoid when creating a gratitude practice.

- **Avoid comparisons.** We may not always notice it, but it's easy to fall into comparison mode when experiencing guilt about expressing gratitude. For instance, you may have had thoughts in the past such as, "Others have it much worse than me" or "At least I'm not as bad off as so-and-so." It's important to remember that your experiences and challenges exist the same as experiences of others and equally worthy of validation and support.

- **Start small.** Start small if you're struggling to think of something you're genuinely grateful for. Maybe you received a funny text from a friend or lit your favorite scented candle, or your homework was more straightforward than you expected. Becoming more aware of even these little things can add up and help you enjoy all the same benefits that come with practicing gratitude more regularly.

- **Be authentic.** Don't try to "fake it till you make it." Sometimes life is hard, and it's okay to acknowledge complicated feelings or situations. It's also okay to not feel grateful all the time. Masking your feelings or pretending to feel grateful when you're not will not serve you in the long run. In fact, it may cause you to experience even more stress.

- **Don't get bogged down.** Some people may find it helpful to keep up a dedicated practice of journaling or letter-writing. However, if these exercises make you feel stressed, practicing gratitude more informally is fine. Finding an approach that works for you long term is more important than creating the "perfect routine."

- **Access resources.** Look at the EDS Society's Toolkit for mental health at https://www.ehlers-danlos.com/mental-health-resources/.

Maintaining a gratitude journal has many benefits, including gaining more energy, feeling more optimistic about life, and possessing better physical and mental health. Its many positive benefits compound to bring you overall better quality of life. Start your own gratitude journal today and see the difference it can make in your life. It sounds simple or even silly, but it can make a big difference when you focus on what you have versus what you lack.

Choose to Assess, Act, or Affirm

- **Assess:** What are three ways you can reduce stress in your life after reading this chapter?
- **Act:** Put a reminder in your phone to do one of those things.
- **Affirm:** "I will find gratitude in something every day."

Bibliography

Martin, S. (n.d.). "10 Stress Management Tips for Busy, Overwhelming, and Stressful Times." Sharon Martin: Live Well and Love Your Life. https://www.livewellwithsharonmartin.com/stress-management/

"Stress in America™ 2020: A National Mental Health Crisis." (2020). *American Psychological Association.* Accessed December 7, 2021. https://www.apa.org/news/press/releases/stress/2020/report-october.

NOTES

CHAPTER 8

MANAGING AUTONOMIC DYSFUNCTION

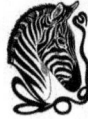

Sometimes you just have to let go of your tight grip of how things should be or how quickly they should come together and simply let things run their own course. By releasing control and letting the currents carry you along, paradoxically, you gain more control of your attitude and your response to what's happening to you at the moment.

—Keri Olson

As human beings, all of our knowledge, experiences, and understanding in life are gathered through our senses – a complex and automatic processing system that alerts us when we are hot or cold, hungry or thirsty, safe or in danger. All day and night our brains are taking in information about the world around us that helps us function in everyday life. Good sensory feedback gives our bodies data to calibrate vital systems including heart rate, sweating, and breathing. However, if the sensory system isn't functioning properly, we can become either hypersensitive or under-sensitive, also known as neurodiversity. Bright lights, ordinary noise levels, or even just clothing touching the skin can cause us to feel overwhelmed.

It is widely recognized that we have five senses: sight, sound, taste, smell, and touch. But there are additional systems of cues that are of particular interest to a hypermobile patient. Proprioception tells us where our bodies are in space (you may be clumsy), vestibular balance helps with posture (you might walk into things), and interoception guides us in dealing with internal regulation responses (the need to go to the bathroom). These systems all culminate in our complete autonomic nervous system (ANS), which can be altered by hEDS.

Our ANS is driven by our involuntary and unconscious minds, meaning we do not have any active control over them. They oversee many of the body's functions, including body temperature, blood pressure, and digestion. Things out of your control such as brain fog and other cognitive issues due to lack of blood flow to the brain (for example, salivation) are also regulated by the ANS. Thank goodness we don't have to consciously think about telling our body to do all of that work!

For those with EDS, it is crucial to understand how the two ANS systems—the sympathetic and parasympathetic—work with each other and how they regulate our behavior. In particular, research led by Dr. Stephen Porges has emerged into developing the polyvagal theory of how humans respond to stress. These systems are responsible for what you might know as the fight, flight, or freeze response.

Understanding the autonomic nervous system

Porges theorized that the fundamental reaction of all animals is involuntary and activated by the sympathetic nervous system when we are threatened, scared, or even startled. It is anything that challenges us and/or what we protect. These are purely defensive strategies to survive, activated by our body, which chooses whether to fight, fly, freeze, or fawn depending on the information we perceive. Peter Levine says in his book *Waking the Tiger* that animals that appear dead will not be eaten by other animals. It is a survival response innate to us as animals. These can also be trauma reactions. I was initially asked by the dysautonomia cardiologist after he saw my test results if I was a trauma survivor. My body was in a hyper-adrenal state of complete overreaction like it had been fighting a war for decades.

The parasympathetic nervous system is the alter ego—the quiet, connected side of us key to interrelating to others and our bonding needs. Like primitive pack animals, we must connect to others. When the parasympathetic nervous system is in charge, we can be both alert and chill. We can live, work, cooperate, and build relationships. The sympathetic nervous system has to be calm for us to operate in the more advanced human state of the parasympathetic nervous system. The former is always alert for stress and danger and can take over at a moment's notice or be affected when we face long-term chronic stress. It will shut down the parasympathetic system completely. It can also impair or prevent healing.

Although the sympathetic system is totally automatic, that doesn't mean it is entirely out of our control. If our brain is unregulated, it can cause our body to go into chaos. Our minds can get us in trouble by simply thinking things and getting us into a physical panic (think of this simply as "worrying yourself sick"). This area of research is expanding and holds the basics of neuroplasticity and retraining our brains to respond in new and different ways to stress responses.

It is critical to learn coping skills and stress management to reduce the reactive nature of our sympathetic nervous system and allow the parasympathetic system to engage. All of your life experiences culminate into your physiological state by adapting to your previous circumstances. Thus, stress and trauma can lead to disease. This is why we need to learn how to manage our autonomic system and its occasional hyper-adrenal overdrive, which is heavily influenced when you have dysautonomia or POTS. It is vital to regain control over your ANS to allow the healing your body naturally knows how to do to begin.

Dysautonomia and EDS

Dysautonomia (also known as autonomic dysfunction) is a general term used to describe various diseases or failures of the ANS and the vagus nerve. Dysautonomia can be a primary disorder, or it can transpire in combination with another condition (such as diabetes) as a secondary disorder. Although the cause of dysautonomia is not known, some think it might be genetic while others believe it could be caused by several different external events—everything from pregnancy, viral illness, and autoimmune disorders to physical trauma, degenerative neurological diseases, and brain injury.

Postural orthostatic tachycardia syndrome (POTS), a type of dysautonomia common in hEDS, refers to an exaggerated increase in heart rate upon standing. When a person goes from lying down to sitting or standing upright, POTS can cause chronic, daily orthostatic symptoms because nearly half a liter of blood moves to the lower extremities (legs, arms, hands, feet), causing a temporary reduction in blood flow to the brain. Typically, these changes activate the ANS, leading to a short-term increase in heart rate.

The sympathetic nerves within the ANS activate the body's fight-or-flight response, including increases in heart rate and blood pressure; the parasympathetic nerves stimulate the "rest-and-digest" response, including decreases in heart rate and blood pressure. In people with POTS, however, something goes wrong with the body's response to upright posture, and they suffer from an excessive increase in heart rate, called tachycardia.

Individuals with hypermobility often have autonomic abnormalities, typically postural tachycardia syndrome, where there is enhanced cardiovascular reactivity and overlap with a potential sensation of having an anxiety disorder. Hypermobile patients are up to 16 times more likely to have panic and anxiety disorders, which is yet to be fully understood. Evidence in medical research suggests a link between hypermobility and stress-sensitive medical disorders. One study in 2012 even says that hypermobile people have a different brain structure including a larger than average amygdala.

Hear from a dysautonomia expert

I had the privilege to interview the co-founder and president of Dysautonomia International Lauren Stiles.[4] Lauren is the co-founder of the global nonprofit overseeing funding of research and education on autonomic nerve disorders. They developed the first postural orthostatic tachycardia syndrome (POTS) patient registry with over 6,000 patients enrolled.

I understand that you have a POTS diagnosis yourself. Tell me your story.

- "After about nine months searching for answers following a snowboarding concussion injury, I figured out myself that I had POTS. I brought the idea to my doctors, and they confirmed that I met

---

[4] For the full transcript, including details on three promising avenues in the current research they are funding, please go to my website at www.holdingitalltogether.com using the password "ZebraStrong!" to access them.

the POTS criteria. But very quickly when I read up on POTS, I realized that POTS was always caused by something else. In many people, we can't identify that something else. But in some cases, we can actually figure out the underlying cause. In my case, the underlying cause was Sjögren's syndrome, which is an autoimmune disease. It is the second most common cause of dysautonomia, the first being diabetes. Sjögren's is the number one autoimmune cause of dysautonomia, and it can cause all the symptoms of POTS and potentially many other problems with various organs and other neurological issues. It is very common in EDS patients as well."

What are the primary goals for the organization?

- "We seek to raise as much money as possible to support research that really matters to our patient community. We're focused on high-impact research designed to deliver more effective treatments... I would love it if we could figure out dysautonomia, how to get rid of it and how to prevent it! Then we wouldn't have to exist as an organization. But that's going to take a long time. In 2022, we celebrate our 10-year anniversary. Some doctors in this field will tell you we have completely transformed the way the medical profession thinks about POTS. When I was diagnosed in 2010, the party line from most doctors, including some experts, was that POTS was 'deconditioning and anxiety in young women.' Now there's a growing understanding that there are tangible neurological deficits, immune dysregulation, and autoimmune going on in a majority of POTS patients, including in the EDS/POTS patients. We're funding research that is exploring these concepts and trying to understand them better so that we can make immune targeted therapies available to these patients."

I know you're researching long Covid, and maybe we're getting a little bit more attention in the mainstream media with symptoms of long Covid being similar to being diagnosed as POTS. Tell me about that research.

- "Wearing my Stony Brook Research Assistant Professor of Neurology hat, and my Dysautonomia International hat, I collaborated with Dr. Mitch Miglis, an autonomic neurologist at Stanford, to study autonomic dysfunction in long Covid. We found that more than a majority of long Covid patients have moderate to severe autonomic dysfunction. It can present as POTS but can also present as other autonomic disorders like orthostatic intolerance or orthostatic hypotension. Long Covid itself is not all POTS or dysautonomia. But a large percentage of what we're calling long

Covid is a classic post-viral dysautonomia. There is so much funding now from the US and European governments, private funders, and even pharma interested in long Covid. What we are trying to do as an organization is encourage those researchers to not only screen for long Covid, but when enrolling long Covid patients into their study, to also screen them for POTS, and orthostatic intolerance, screen them for EDS and chronic fatigue, and report out the data on these different cohorts. There's literally been over a billion dollars that Congress gave for long Covid to date. Just for comparison, cancer doesn't get that much money."

What medical research is going on now to help POTS and EDS patients funded by DI?

- "About one-third of POTS patients have hypermobile EDS. There's an often-repeated myth in our patient community that EDS causes POTS because it gives you floppy blood vessels that cause blood pooling when EDS patients stand up. That could be true, but we actually have no research that explores this. So we have been pushing researchers to study this—to ask if POTS patients who have EDS are biologically different than POTS patients who don't have EDS. We know that all POTS patients tend to pool blood in their lower abdominal area and limbs when they stand up, whether they have EDS or not. What we need to explore is, is that caused by a different mechanism in the POTS/EDS patients than the POTS/no EDS patients? Is it the same mechanism, but perhaps just made a little worse by the EDS? We don't actually know. So we're trying to answer these questions with our research funding. There are a lot of theories, but we don't have a lot of data. Patients deserve real answers based on credible research, not a guess. We really need to make sure that that research happens so that our patients are given accurate information. The more we understand about the biology of why EDS and POTS overlap, the more precise we can be in develop new treatments that treat the root causes of these disorders."

I know that Dysautonomia International has a great deal of resources, but what do you think is the best patient resource that you offer to the dysautonomia community?

- "I think for patients and caregivers who want to learn about this in depth and the correlation of EDS, POTS, MCAS, and autoimmunity, the best resource we offer is our Autonomic Disorders Video Library, located at www.vimeo.com/dysautonomia. You can also get to it through our main website, www.dysautonomiainternational.org. We have over 190 educational videos and lectures from the top experts in all of these conditions, the top EDS experts, the top dysautonomia experts, the top mast cell experts. Each of those lectures goes in depth about what we know and what we don't know, where the current research is headed, what are the standard treatments, and what are the cutting-edge treatments. It's a great resource for patients—and for their doctors."

What to avoid and what can help

A few things can worsen my POTS symptoms in particular, which are common for POTS patients in general. Standing (or sitting) for a long time is a trigger, but so are low-pressure weather fronts. Any significant change in the barometric pressure can leave me feeling horrible. I watch my barometer and use an app (Weather X) to warn me of any impending weather changes such as an impending thunderstorm. Other things include hot and humid days, which make it easier to get lightheaded when it's warm outside, especially if I am dehydrated. Not enough salt, too much caffeine, or a spike in my blood sugar has a similar effect—my blood vessels enlarge, leading to increased blood pooling in my feet and legs.

However, since POTS can occur for different reasons for different people, it typically comes down to the individual. In my case not eating enough nutritious, protein-packed food and/or eating processed foods that are harder to digest is a trigger, as is focusing on a computer or phone screen too long. Viral illnesses such as colds or the flu, anxiety and depression, and even sexual activity can cause it to flare.

POTS patients should generally avoid some activities, but make sure you discuss these with your practitioners because not all POTS patients are the same.

- Extreme heat;
- Getting dehydrated;
- Caffeine (especially energy drinks);
- Extra-large meals;
- Alcohol;
- Foods high in gluten or other allergens;
- Donating blood;
- Standing up quickly or for long periods;
- Holding arms up for an extended time;
- Stressful work environments;
- Lifting objects over 10–15 pounds;
- Climbing long flights of stairs.

The bottom line is you must learn to listen to your body. Keep a symptom journal and write down what makes you feel better or worse, so you know what to do if you have a terrible episode. And if you are a friend/family member of a POTS patient, be willing to let some things go and think outside of the box regarding daily activities and how you might help out. Learn about the triggers for the POTS sufferer in your world, and help them stay clear of the things to avoid.

People can better manage POTS symptoms with specific body postures and physical maneuvers. For example, when upright, contracting muscles to pump blood back to the heart and compress the abdomen to reduce blood pooling in the intestinal circulation can help relieve symptoms. Even a slight increase in the blood return to the heart can help maintain an adequate blood flow to the brain. Lying down flat is best, but when you can't, try these positions:

- Standing with legs crossed;
- Squatting;
- Standing with one leg on a chair;
- Bending forward from the waist (such as leaning over a shopping cart);
- Sitting in the knee-chest position;
- Sitting in a low chair with feet raised;
- Leaning forward with hands on the knees when sitting.

Another huge positive impact you can have on POTS is exercise and movement, but that deserves its own chapter. Overall, the day-to-day management of most types of EDS, including hEDS, revolves around the right kind of physical therapy, exercise, and (it turns out) pacing.

Pacing yourself

What I mean by pacing is giving yourself the grace to know when to pause or stop. This not only applies to POTS patients but to all of us with EDS. We don't often realize or feel it when we have overdone it until it's too late. In truth I wouldn't go anywhere without the ability to charge my cell phone. So why would I allow my body to be depleted and run out of energy?

Learning how to pace yourself can be difficult but well worth the effort to better balance your energy and reduce recovery time from overdoing it. I am the queen of overdoing it, and this lesson is hard for me to put into practice because like many with EDS I want to be able to do what normal people can do—go for walks, take exciting vacations, or even just withstand long doctor appointments.

The notion of pacing is sometimes pictured in terms of "spoons" (everyone only has so many spoons per day to use up) or even "recharging a bad cell phone battery theory" (the battery is inconsistent and some days charges okay and other days the battery runs out of juice quickly). However you envision your energy stores, it's important that you understand how your actions can draw them down and how you can save a spoon or recharge your batteries before you realize you're cooked and well done. Try not to get caught in the cycle of boom, bust, and burnout.

One unique approach to pacing is through the eyes of Hannah Ensore, founder of Stickman Communications. She developed a visual way to help others understand EDS and its challenges using simple illustrations. She describes pacing as "the way of getting the most from the energy you have. It is commonly used for conditions that cause persistent pain or fatigue." One of her key insightful products is a book and activity decision chart on pacing.

She teaches you how to not push through symptoms causing them to get worse but to recognize what activities make it worse and what exactly can help to create a lifestyle that works for you. Her *To Do or Not to Do* decision chart has helped me better decide what I should and not do on a regular basis.

Choose to Assess, Act, or Affirm

- **Assess:** Have you experienced dysautonomia symptoms, including dizziness, loss of balance, racing heart? Do you feel faint when you stand?

- **Act:** Try this 60-second test at home: Hold one hand over your head, the other below your waist while standing. Hold for 30 seconds. Release both hands and bring to the center of your body near your waistline. Do your hands look different? Blood flow is affected if you have POTS and can cause changes in the color of your hands.

- **Affirm:** "I treat my discomfort and pain like I would an innocent child. I tend to my body with unconditional compassion and care."

Bibliography

Eccles, J. A., Beacher, F. D., Gray, M. A., Jones, C. L., Minati, L., Harrison, N. A., and Critchley, H. D. (2012). "Brain Structure and Joint Hypermobility: Relevance to the Expression of Psychiatric Symptoms." *The British Journal of Psychiatry*, 200(6), 508–509. https://doi.org/10.1192/bjp.bp.111.092460

Ensore, H. *The Pocket Book of Pacing*. Stickman Communications, Inc. https://stickmancommunications.co.uk/product/the-pocket-book-of-pacing/.

Garcia Campayo J, Asso E, Alda M, Andres EM, Sobradiel N. (2010). "Association between Joint Hypermobility Syndrome and Panic Disorder: a Case–Control Study." *Psychosomatics* 51:55–61.

Frederick, A., and Levine, P. *Waking the Tiger: Healing Trauma: The Innate Capacity to Transform Overwhelming Experiences*. North Atlantic Books, 1997.

Porges, S. W. (2009). "The Polyvagal Theory: New Insights into Adaptive Reactions of the Autonomic Nervous System." *Cleve Clin J Med.* 76(Suppl 2): S86–S90. https://www.ncbi.nlm.nih.gov/pmc/articles/PMC3108032/.

NOTES

CHAPTER 9

MINDFULNESS AND MEDITATION

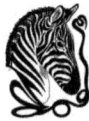

Write a to-be list, instead of a to-do list, for tomorrow. It may look something like this: Tomorrow, I will be mindful, aware, peaceful, a person who seeks reasons to smile and laugh, loving, appreciative, forgiving, thoughtful, supportive, still, quiet, faithful, honest, a person who simply wants to be. The quality of your life is determined by who you are, not by what you accomplish. We are, after all, human beings, not human doings. Let's base the value of our day on that small bit of wisdom and live accordingly. Just be.

—Nancy Daley

---

believe that finding a way to calm the chaos of our everyday lives is imperative. I also believe that relaxation is a skill. Unwinding the monkey mind and resetting your thought patterns is the key to stress reduction and improving your coping skills to help you face your chronic illness. Among the many different ways you can learn to relax, mindfulness and meditation have recently gone more mainstream and become widely accepted forms of self-regulation. I wholeheartedly believe in their power to change your mind and body for the better as both had the most profound impact on my overall healing. In fact, the more I learned about them, the more convinced I became till I eventually became trained and certified to teach them. The best part is they are available anytime, anywhere, for free!

Stress reduction is achievable with regular mindfulness practice and meditation. While learning mindfulness and how to meditate is not easy, they are habits you can learn to master. Learning about mindfulness and meditation changed my state of being for the better—so much better. This chapter will take the "woo-woo" out of both topics and provide practical, simple tools to help you change your life for the better too.

Mindfulness and meditation basics

Our minds are racing all the time—so much so that to force a slow down seems impossible despite the fact we crave rest so much. But with the help of mindfulness and meditation, I managed to recondition myself to slow down and smell the roses. I firmly believe in the power of becoming more present through mindfulness because I believe the practice quite literally saved my life.

Wendy Quan of The Calm Monkey (the mindfulness training company where I obtained my certification) explained the similarities and differences between mindfulness and meditation to me this way:

> **Mindfulness** is the practice of being "present" and "in the now" with less judgment and with kindness. You can catch yourself anytime during your day and give your full, quality attention to what you are experiencing in the present moment. Elements of this practice include using your body's five senses to anchor you, noticing and acknowledging your reactions and emotions, and not judging what's happening in a good or a bad way. It's about moment-to-moment awareness.

> **Meditation** is the practice of concentrating on the "object" of the meditation (i.e., your breath, a mantra, a visualization). It is not about having a blank mind and is not necessarily religious. There are many different kinds of meditation, including guided visualizations and open awareness as well as seated versus moving meditations like yoga, walking, and tai chi. Meditation is hitting the pause button during the day and carving out some time to refocus your mind.

> **Mindfulness meditation** is performing a meditation that keeps you in the present moment. A good example is when you are meditating on your breath, meaning that your breath is the object or focus of your

meditation that keeps you in the present moment. A guided visualization such as walking along a sandy beach would not be a mindful meditation.

Key traits of mindfulness

According to The Calm Monkey, the key traits of mindfulness include the following:

- **Presence:** "Being in the now" as often as you can as you go about your day. Mindfulness is bringing full attention to what you are experiencing in the present moment and not thinking about the past or the future.

- **Awareness:** Being self-aware of what you are experiencing within you and around you. (i.e., observing your thoughts, emotions, and body's sensations and what is around you, such as other people's body language, objects around you, etc.).

- **Non-judgment:** Not getting caught up in our stream of likes and dislikes but seeing things as they actually are. It's not very practical to be entirely rid of all judgments, but we can become more aware of our tendency to judge. Accepting reality does *not* mean we have to like the way things are or passively resign ourselves to them. It simply means having a willingness to observe what is happening and the acceptance that it is happening so we don't get stuck and can move forward with intention.

- **Compassion and kindness**: This is about acting with kindness toward ourselves and others. When we have self-talk and deal with other people, it's good to check in with ourselves before we speak by asking whether what we are going to say is kind, helpful, and true.

By practicing mindfulness, we become much more aware of how we live our lives. We stop operating on auto-pilot and live life more consciously. Life begins to have more meaning. We realize that the number of accomplishments doesn't necessarily equate to happiness. We become aware of what is important. We may be able to see why we tend

WHAT HELPED MY UNDERSTANDING OF MINDFULNESS

The goal of "pure" mindfulness is *not* changing one's state of being (like transforming sadness into happiness). Mindfulness instead is about allowing yourself to be with your thoughts and whatever sensations occur, whether we deem them as pleasant or unpleasant, and not judging them or trying to take action on them. That's not to say that an outcome of practicing mindfulness could lead to a conscious decision to make a change. But the kind of change we would make would be one guided by the principles of kindness and truth and based on seeing the world as it is.

to strive and realize that we cannot solve the world's problems by overdoing things to our detriment.

My invitation to you is to begin practicing mindfulness. Think about opportunities and occasions in your own life where you can practice these principles. If we are positively touching humanity, we are making a difference by being here. And we can create a better life experience for ourselves by living more consciously.

The mind-body connection

Mindfulness and meditation work by engaging your parasympathetic nervous system, which essentially turns on your body's natural ability to heal. Your vagus nerve serves as the on/off switch to activate your parasympathetic nervous system. This complex sensory cranial nerve starts at the base of the brain and travels down each side of your neck through your stomach and abdomen, energizing your heart and lungs and connecting your neck, throat, ear, and face muscles.

Activating any of the multiple organs innervated by your vagus nerve can help stimulate it to activate your parasympathetic nervous system and help heal those processes controlled by the organ. Stimulating each of these organs can benefit you in different ways:

- **Brain**, which helps calm inflammation, control anxiety, and relieve depression;
- **Tongue**, which helps to improve taste and saliva production, swallowing, and speech;

- **Ears,** which help to ease tinnitus;
- **Eyes,** which help pupils make eye contact and promote social connection and safety;
- **Larynx,** which helps feed your lungs and diaphragm with oxygen;
- **Stomach,** which helps to stimulate stomach acid for healthy digestion;
- **Intestines,** which allow for nutrient absorption and trigger muscle contractions (peristalsis) to allow food and waste to move through the digestive tract;
- **Pancreas,** which triggers the production and release of enzymes that aid in digestion;
- **Liver,** which triggers detoxification and supports blood sugar functions;
- **Lungs,** which allow your airways to expand and contract;
- **Gallbladder,** which triggers the release of bile that rids the body of toxins and breaks down fat (critical for most paleo and keto diets);
- **Heart,** which helps to regulate heart rate and blood pressure;
- **Spleen,** which inhibits inflammation by calming the release of proinflammatory cytokines (substances secreted by inflammatory cells that affect other cells);
- **Kidney,** which releases sodium, increases blood flow, and manages blood sugar;

- **Bladder,** which allows for retention to prevent frequent urination;
- **Reproductive organs and genitals,** which support fertility and sexual arousal;
- **Immune system,** which regulates inflammation, switching off the production of proteins that fuel the inflammatory immune response.

The following practices shared by Jodie Cohen at Vibrant Blue Oils engage these areas of the mind-body feedback loop to enhance and stimulate the healthy functioning of your vagus nerve to activate your parasympathetic state, which will enhance healing and calm your stress response. Her website (www.vibrantblueoils.com) has great resources on stimulating your vagus nerve to calm your nervous system (including her custom oil called Parasympathetic blend):

- Splash cold water on your face or neck;
- Paint the roof of your mouth with your tongue;
- Massage your neck near the carotid artery gently;
- Take deep diaphragmatic breaths;
- Try sleeping on your right side;
- Get some sunlight;
- Support a healthy gut;
- Hum, sing, or chant, especially while exhaling.

The goal of these polyvagal stimulating exercises is to reduce your fight-flight response systems. We can teach our bodies to stop reacting to simple things such as traffic as if it were a raging bear threatening us. Those suffering from chronic illness are also in a chronic state of stress, but you can unlearn that behavior. You can teach your brain and your body through mindfulness and meditation to dampen or even stop the fight-or-flight response.

The benefits of meditation

Meditation has a long history of use for increasing calmness and physical relaxation, improving psychological balance, coping with illness, and enhancing overall health and well-being. The list of benefits that people often get from meditation is tangible, such as stress reduction, reduced anxiety, better decision-making, increased gratitude, and more joy.

But there's a reason that we now regularly hear about the health benefits of meditation or hear about the famous athletes, celebrities, or business leaders who rely on the practice: Over the last forty years, we have witnessed a revolution in research on this ancient practice. At last count, over 6,000 peer-reviewed scholarly articles have been published that examine the subject. This vast body of neuroscience research has found that the regular practice of meditation leads to the following benefits:

- *Increased resilience:* Meditation is associated with a reduction in activity in the part of the brain that reacts to stress. This enhances our ability to stay calm and responsive during stressful situations.

- *Increased focus:* Meditation activates additional circuits in the brain that allow for sharper and more efficient concentration.

- *Decreased mind wandering:* Meditation reduces moments when our attention wanders away from what is happening here and now.

- *Enhanced pain tolerance:* Mindfulness triggers a neurological, pain-relieving response.

- *Enhanced immunity:* Meditation has been found to reduce markers of inflammation in the body and strengthen the immune system's response.

Many studies have reviewed the benefits of meditation for different conditions. According to a health summary of research on meditation from the National Institutes of Health (https://www.nccih.nih.gov/health/meditation-in-depth), there is evidence that it may reduce blood pressure as well as symptoms of irritable bowel syndrome and flare-ups in people who have had ulcerative colitis. The Harvard Health research article *Understanding Depression* notes that meditation has "distinct effects on the brain" and, in turn, the rest of the body, calming the stress response and reducing the risk associated with high blood pressure. There is also research indicating that meditation may ease symptoms of anxiety and depression and help people with insomnia.

For example, many people with chronic diseases wake up anxious in the morning (because cortisol spikes then). Individuals with higher levels of anxiety may not get as much restorative sleep. The ongoing stress (without respite) is what can lead to that feeling of panic when your alarm clock sounds. In his article, "3 Reasons You're More Anxious in the Morning (And How to Fix It)," Dominique Astorino noted that mornings (and especially Monday mornings) are considered prime time for heart attacks for this same reason. Research published in 2018 by the NIH shows "the occurrence of stroke, myocardial infarction, and sudden cardiac death all have daily patterns, striking most frequently in the morning." But you can counter the effects of this by practicing mindfulness before bed through (for example) an evening breathing practice routine. This can help alleviate the unknown and calm the potential chaos that can spike autonomic dysfunction.

Research about meditation's ability to reduce pain has produced mixed results. However, in some studies, scientists suggest that meditation activates certain brain areas in response to pain. A small 2016 study funded in part by the National Center for Complementary and Integrative Health (NCCIH) found that mindfulness meditation does help to control pain while not using the brain's naturally occurring opiates to do so. This suggests that combining mindfulness with pain medications and other approaches that rely on the brain's opioid activity may be particularly effective for reducing pain.

Studies have found meditation affects markers of inflammation (C-reactive protein), which in higher levels can harm one's physical health. Research shows that people with rheumatoid arthritis have reduced C-reactive protein levels after taking a mindfulness-based stress reduction (MBSR) course. Overall, these findings suggest that mindfulness meditation can have disease-fighting powers through our immune response.

One of the essential benefits that leads to resilience is learning how to respond and not react (essentially meaning overreact), which is very typical for hyper-reactive chronically ill patients. When something occurs, we sometimes immediately begin to allow our minds to catastrophize before we've absorbed it. Because of the constant challenges and dangers we face, this kind of thinking is common for those with EDS and even might feel like it's become hard-wired into how we think. But we can train ourselves to think differently and teach ourselves not to react. With time we come to understand through "pure" mindfulness about "being with what it is," including being with and accepting the reality of the state of your chronic illness and the challenges and opportunities it provides you.

Physical pain is not only felt in the body; our thoughts, feelings, and emotional reactions influence our experience of chronic pain. Struggling against these normal stress-pain reactions can leave us feeling helpless and contribute to making the pain worse. Mindfulness practices can help separate pain from the judgment that affects how we experience it. If you are interested in calming your pain through mindfulness, I recommend the Curable app, which teaches you how to get your thoughts changed around your pain.

HOW MINDFUL MEDITATION MAY HELP CHRONIC PAIN

Mindfulness can not only keep us calmer and in the present moment but can also change the shape of our brain and alleviate pain. Watch the video of Erin who suffers from pain associated with multiple sclerosis. After practicing mindful meditation for eight weeks, her pain had improved, and MRIs revealed actual changes to structures in her brain. These groundbreaking studies show that mindfulness can affect networks in our brain that we previously thought we had no control over. Check it out here on YouTube:

https://www.youtube.com/watch?v=4gNFXuiMrck

Mindful meditation isn't just for improving the lives of those with chronic illness. Every single one of us experiences pain and suffering, and we all see it all around us. Trauma, grief, tragedy, illness, loss—these are all unavoidable parts of being human. Even those who experience less hardship than most still have to watch the people they love struggle at times, wishing we could somehow help. Mindfulness teaches us we can, and that it's far more straightforward than we may think. We don't need to save people, fix their problems, or change their lives. We just need to care and be there for them with open arms and ears and a loving, compassionate heart. Mindfulness can help cultivate that spirit within us. When we think better and feel better, life becomes a different experience altogether.

I'm interested in trying meditation, but how do I start?

You know that meditation is more than just sitting quietly, so the next logical question you may still be asking yourself is, "How do I do it?"

First, you need to take some steps to prepare to meditate.

> *Find a quiet place.* It is helpful to have a designated area where you can meditate. There's something about the energy of a space that matters. The energy becomes a support mechanism. I use a specific chair because I like to think of it as a giant oak tree that I'm leaning against in nature, and I'm being supported entirely by the tree that's been there for hundreds of years before me and will be hundreds of years after me.

> *Start small.* It is best to be undisturbed for whatever amount of time you decide. Start small, perhaps with just a few minutes, maybe even just five, gradually increasing to what feels comfortable.

> *A place to be still.* This can be a cushion, chair, or even a bed, if that fosters relaxation but not sleep. You can meditate standing up. You can meditate lying down or any way you want.

Sound. While not required, sound can provide another way to keep unwanted thoughts at bay. Plenty of YouTube videos and phone apps provide free access to soothing tones, ranging from running water Himalayan singing bowls to Tibetan sound bowls if you're into that. Try Spotify playlists for vagal tone. What is most important is that you have a quiet space and that the sound is either something you're focusing on purposefully or that is completely quiet, and you try to remain distraction-free.

Once you are comfortable with your when and where, the basic instructions for focused attention meditation are as follows:

- Sit with a straight spine, eyes preferably closed or in a downward gaze. Proper sitting posture is encouraged to help you stay present and alert rather than relaxed. (Remember, the purpose is to be alert and present, not rest and move into sleep!)

- Bring your attention to the sensations of breathing (either at your nose or in your chest or abdomen). Breathing allows you to sense the present moment, and it is a great tool to bring your consciousness back to the present if you are ever caught in your thoughts.

- When the mind wanders, notice that you are thinking, then shift your attention back to the breath, and stay with each inhale and exhale. Shift your focus again and again as you get distracted or caught up in thought. Being aware of every moment and at that moment will allow you to embrace the present moment, no matter what comes with it (therein lies acceptance, often the most challenging part).

With so many different meditation techniques offered by an expansive list of providers and its popularity becoming more mainstream, it's easy to get overwhelmed. To narrow down which methods may be best for you, start by asking yourself if you want to be guided through your meditation by someone else or if you prefer to be your own guide. Guided meditation is a great place to begin your practice if you're brand-new, as it will help you learn which types of meditations you enjoy and benefit from the most (that is what the popular Calm app provides). They can also help you learn how to do biofeedback and meditate so that you can eventually practice on your own.

Once you determine how you want your meditation led, consider what outcome you want to obtain from your meditation practice. Do you want a meditation that focuses on making you calmer and at peace, or a meditation that may help you learn more about yourself? If you're going to focus on reducing symptoms of stress and feeling calmer, start your search for reflections that encourage you to find calm by focusing on one thing (your breath, a mantra, or a sound). If you want to learn more about yourself, try a practice that involves bringing your awareness to the more nuanced aspects of who you are physically, mentally, and emotionally (consider a loving kindness meditation). Once you've determined how you want to practice and what you want to get out of meditation, you can further your research on specific types of meditation techniques.

THE QUICK START METHOD: A MINI MEDITATION

Start by shifting your attention to your breath. Without altering your breath pattern at all, notice *how* you're breathing. Where does the breath enter (your nostrils or your mouth)? and how does it feel flowing in and out of your body?

Now, take a much deeper breath through your nose. Let it linger for a brief moment, then let your breath exit through your mouth. Repeat three to five more times at your own pace.

Do you feel any different? Perhaps you feel less tired, stressed, or anxious? Maybe you're not sure what you think, and that's perfectly valid too. If something arises—sensations, emotions, thoughts—whatever it might be that is strong enough to take your attention away from the feeling of the breath, or if you've fallen asleep, or you get lost in some incredible fantasy, see if you can let go and begin again, bringing your attention back to the breath. If you have to let go and start a thousand times again, it's okay—that's the practice. That is meditation.

Finally, remember to identify a convenient time and place to meditate. If you're new to meditation, you can try starting with as little as one minute of meditation each day and then build up slowly to longer practice sessions. As with most things in life, you are developing, and benefitting from a mediation practice takes time. That's why they call it a meditation *practice*. The more consistent you are with your meditation, the more you will benefit.

Respiration is an unconscious activity of the body, meaning we don't have to think about it for our bodies to do it. Though it's an involuntary process, breathing can have a powerful effect on our physical and mental health, and it can also be an indicator of underlying health issues. Breathing patterns that indicate a stressful or anxious state include short, and shallow inhales and irregular breaths. These breathing patterns can prolong these feelings of stress or anxiety. But breathing isn't just an indicator of how you are feeling—it's also a tool you can use to manage these symptoms of stress and anxiety and handle them better.

While the breath can be a powerful tool to help ease symptoms of stress and anxiety, sometimes breathing isn't enough. If you are experiencing extreme or persistent feelings of stress, anxiety, or depression, I encourage you to seek help from a licensed mental health care professional.

Choose to Assess, Act, or Affirm

- **Assess:** Have you ever tried mindfulness or meditation practices consistently? What good benefits do you receive from any of the mediTations you are currently taking? How might they have changed your life for the better?

- **Act:** Download and try the Insight Timer free meditation app/website and try it for 7–10 days to see if you notice any changes. Invest in the Calm app for daily or regular practice if you like it.

- **Affirm:** "I can find time for myself and my needs."

Bibliography

Astorino, D. (2021). "3 Reasons You're More Anxious in the Morning (And How To Fix It)." *HuffPost.* https://www.huffingtonpost.co.uk/entry/how-to-fix-morning-anxiety_uk_61606e0de4b019644424aa77.

Cohen, J. (2020). "Essential Oils to Boost the Brain & Heal the Body." https://boostthebrainbook.com/wp-content/uploads/2021/03/VBO_Bonus_Chapter_Jodi_Cohen_2021.pdf.

"Interested in Meditation? Here Are the Basics." (n.d.). *Mindful.* https://www.mindful.org/interested-in-meditation-here-are-the-basics/.

Kabat-Zinn, J. (n.d.). "Everyday Mindfulness with Jon Kabat-Zinn." *Mindful.org.* https://www.mindful.org/everyday-mindfulness-with-jon-kabat-zinn/.

"Meditation." (n.d.). National Center for Complementary and Integrative Health. https://files.nccih.nih.gov/s3fs-public/Meditation_04-25-2016.pdf.

"Meditation: In-Depth" | NCCIH. (n.d.). National Center for Complementary and Integrative Health. https://www.nccih.nih.gov/health/meditation-in-depth.

Understanding Depression. (n.d.). Harvard Health. https://www.health.harvard.edu/mind-and-mood/understanding-depression.

NOTES

PART IV

HEALING HABITS FOR YOUR BODY

In this part I take a deeper dive into the topic of bodily care and what you can do to tend to your body's ever-changing needs. Much of the pain and frustration of hypermobility is rooted in the physical aspects of how your body moves, doesn't move, and how it responds to those movements. If we sublux, dislocate or hyperextend our joints, our muscles and organs get out of whack. Therefore, it is critical to find avenues to successfully care for your body and its unique issues. There are key therapies to engage in including regular movement, monitoring of the meals and nutrients you put into your body, and the strength building and relaxation maneuvers found in physical therapy and massage.

While there is no cure yet for EDS, treatment is just as much about doing the things that help as it is avoiding the things that harm. There is an abundance of treatments for the specific issues that arise from OT/PT to braces, splints, and supports for unstable joints, weak muscles, or faulty nerves to dietary modification or supplements for malabsorption issues and pharmacotherapy for muscle pain or nerve pain. There are many possibilities for management of the physical aspects. In addition, there are many potential medical problems a person with EDS faces, and being aware of them can improve quality of life and quality of treatment. This includes knowing about risks with some antibiotics in the fluoroquinolone family (Cipro, etc.) and special considerations about anesthetics during routine medical care.

While a life with EDS is not going to be as expected for most patients, the knowledge to be able to make better decisions about career choices, family planning, lifestyle, and treatment can make more of these things possible.

CHAPTER 10

MOVEMENT

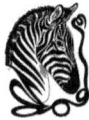

*We often cling to our desires and fight for them
because we think we'll be happy if we get what we
want. But when we let go and accept what is, what
shows up for us are often the things we need.*

—Dezryelle Arcieri

Exercise is important for everyone for many reasons, yet for those with hypermobility, exercise can be key for condition management. The type of movement that will be suitable will depend on how severely you are affected. But in my opinion, if you want to feel better overall, the best thing I can suggest is to move your body—if only for a few minutes daily. It can enhance cardiovascular fitness, alertness, sleep quality, and also improve proprioception, muscle strength, reduce chronic pain, and maximize bone density to reduce potential osteoporosis.

Many patients with EDS can benefit from low-impact exercises, such as rowing, recumbent biking, Pilates, qigong, and tai chi, which help build core strength while being restorative. Gentle restorative style yoga also can be beneficial but poses must be done carefully as there is the risk of overextending joints in some positions. Swimming or any aquatic movement can also be helpful for some EDS patients, which we will dive into (no pun intended) later in this chapter.

Before you begin an exercise regimen to help manage your symptoms, check with your doctor and get cleared to exercise. Your doctor can help you identify your exercise therapy's target heart ranges and goals.

The benefits of movement

Feeling better means making yourself move every day. For me, the more pain I feel, the more I need to move. I know it's easy to say and a different story actually to do. But the payoff is enormous over time. This is the basis of many of the physical therapy protocols such as CHOP, Muldowney, Levine, and others to increase your physical stamina and resilience. It's also good for dysautonomia, according to Dr. Italo Biaggioni at Vanderbilt University, "Movement is the number one way to get out of fight-or-flight."

It's important to know before adding any movement or mild exercise to your routine to start small and stay within the mid-range of motion to avoid hyperextending joints. Manage your expectations of what you can and should do. It is very easy to overdo it because our bodies often don't send us the proper signals that we have done too much until after when it is too late, potentially causing a cycle of overuse, flare, and repeat.

If I had only one word of wisdom to share...try very hard to force yourself to move your body daily. I know it's next to impossible when you're tired, weary, and feeling unstable in the joints. Even a few minutes can really enhance how much better you will feel.

Several different options are available to patients who want to begin an exercise program. You can see a physical therapist, which is a great way to start to learn the types of exercises you should and shouldn't do. Or you can hire a personal trainer to help get you started. If you are home-bound, you may be able to have a personal trainer or physical therapist visit you in the home. You can also work out on your own at home or join a local gym or pool.

When you have EDS and POTS and/or other comorbidities, you are likely to be exercise intolerant, which means you cannot exercise for any period without breathlessness and extreme fatigue. Many of us cannot tolerate the heat of any outdoor activity either. When we can exercise or go on a fun but exerting outing, many will typically flare the next day or maybe for a few days—you pay for it. It's super frustrating! But movement remains the number one way to start the change of momentum to heal: move, feel better, move more, feel even better...

and so on. You will see benefits in as little as two weeks of regular movement.

Remember as well that everyone begins at a different starting point. Where you start with your exercise therapy depends on your current level of fitness. If you have been bedridden for years and cannot walk without mobility aids, you will obviously begin to be slower than someone who works a full-time job or spends time on their feet all day. I started with two to three minutes. And then you just move for a few minutes more than the day before.

However, there is a scale of effort you must pay attention to. If you start out doing two to three minutes of simple walking, recumbent bike, or whatever is your low-impact exercise of choice—don't overdo it! That will put you in a cycle—flare-recover-atrophy-start over—with training required to begin again. Start small and do tiny incremental increases over a more extended time to gain strength and capacity. Soon you will find you are doing a lot more than you believed you could. Start with three to five minutes, then six minutes, then seven minutes, and so on.

The biggest lesson I learned is that if I don't exercise for even as few as two days in a row, I have to start all over again at the bottom. That is how fast you can lose your stamina and physical ability to tolerate exercise. Find an activity you get joy from and make it a part of your daily life as a wellness therapy you choose to do for yourself first.

Types of exercise helpful for hypermobile patients

Although it can be harder for people to find the right exercise program they can tolerate regularly, there are many pathways to try where you can listen to your body and do what works for you. It is recommended to exercise while seated (recumbent) and to focus on your core posture and spinal muscle stability.

Let's be very clear—I'm not talking about engaging in P90X workouts, even for just three minutes. I'm talking about low-impact and gentle exercise. Here are some good options.

Walking: Start simple by trying a daily five-to-ten minute walk—no speed walking or overexertion. If you have a place in nature you can walk, it is even more beneficial to your mindset. I enjoy 15-to-20-minute walks with my dog three to four times a day. Sometimes I go longer, and sometimes I cannot take more than five minutes. Those days of short walks are hard on your spirit, but persevere as the next day will offer another opportunity to move.

Aqua exercise: Swimming or just moving in water is one of the best exercise activities for hypermobile people. The water reduces the gravitational pull on your body, allowing your body to be stable and rest while you move, reducing the risk of subluxation. In fact water fitness may help you recover more quickly from injury. For instance, if you have recently undergone some type of major surgery, water fitness can help you rebuild your muscle strength, which aids in quicker recovery. Water fitness is a unique way of building your physical endurance, and increased strength and capabilities can positively affect self-esteem and mental health.

Recumbent exercise: The third recommended exercise is low-impact movement on machines at home or at the gym that keep you recumbent. By not standing or being fully upright, you keep dysautonomia at bay. I bought a recumbent bike for my home, and I can ride it between three and 20 minutes a day depending on my state of fatigue that particular day.

Dysautonomia International recommends various exercise protocols, including reclined exercises such as stretches, yoga, and gentle weightlifting from seated or lying down and recumbent biking, rowing, and swimming. I do other

WATER AS COMPRESSION

According to Dysautonomia International, doctors often recommend that dysautonomia patients wear medical compression stockings of 20–30 mm Hg strength to counteract the blood pooling many patients experience when they stand up. If you are standing in a 4 ft deep pool, the pressure on your toes is equivalent to wearing 90 mm Hg compression stockings. Pools are like giant compression stockings!

low-impact activities or low to the ground movements such as rowing and simple stretching. Only after you have spent a substantial amount of time building up a tolerance to these exercises should you attempt to begin upright activities such as jogging or upright biking.

Gentle mindful movement practices

I discovered mindful movement practices in tai chi and my favorite, qigong. The benefit of Eastern approaches of mindful movement is powerful in calming and soothing both the mind and the body. I started with a 7-minute qigong routine every day for 30 days to build postural strength. The simple, steady, mindful movements gave me a sense of peace, focus, and intention on very slowly building strength. Building my core and back muscle strength has been remarkable to overall stability.

If you are looking for a program, I highly recommend Lee Holden's online program for qigong practices at https://www.holdenqigong.com/. He is a trained instructor who also recovered from health issues including a broken back. He is inspirational yet straightforward in his guidance.

Practicing qigong also made me interested in learning more about mindfulness, opening a window to the possibility of precious moments of calm through breathing and simple meditation attempts. It sparked my interest in learning more about breathing practices to calm the ANS to halt my fight-or-flight over-reactivity.

Choose to Assess, Act, or Affirm

- **Assess:** Are there any types of exercise that your body can tolerate now?
- **Act:** Add a ten-minute walk or other new activity on most days to your routine, preferably outdoors if you can.
- **Affirm:** "I can do hard things."

Bibliography

Dysautonomia International. (n.d.). "Exercises for Dysautonomia Patients." http://www.dysautonomiainternational.org/page.php?ID=43.

NOTES

CHAPTER 11

MEALS AND MINERALS

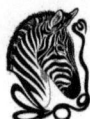

---

*No matter who you are, what you do, and which part
of the world you want to see. If you want a reason to
complain, you will find many things around you that
aren't right. If you seek happiness, you will notice
many parts of your life that are a reason to rejoice.*

—**Maxim D'Souza**

Fueling your body

One of the most essential things when considering how
you fuel your body with good meals and good nutrients
is ensuring your gastrointestinal system is working properly. Many EDSers have gastrointestinal issues in some
form. Doctors often diagnose irritable bowel syndrome
(IBS) before EDS is discovered. The bottom line boils

down to this: Your immune system starts in the gut. Get thorough examinations and do colon and endoscopy tests to rule out other things with a gastroenterologist.

Many years ago, I was diagnosed with leaky gut by a naturopath. I took probiotics for years to heal gut issues that are now mostly in balance. If you have problems with your GI system, you might need to get tested for celiac disease and consider an elimination diet such as going gluten-free. I have found it beneficial to go gluten-free and feel much better. Give it a try and see how your body responds.

When I am exposed to gluten after being gluten-free for so long (which I call "getting glutened"), it makes me terribly sick. My entire GI system is wrecked for days, and I sometimes get hives, swelling in my lips, and am overcome with fatigue. It's a quick reminder of why I eat no gluten by choice.

Many people also see improvements in their symptoms when they eliminate dairy or sugar/sucrose from their diet. Dairy products such as cheese and full-fat cow's milk contain saturated fat, and saturated fat can increase inflammation in the body. Some people see improvements in chronic constipation issues, bloating, gas, and even their energy levels.

You might also consider doing some research about an anti-inflammatory diet that involves removing sugar from your diet. When you eat too much sugar, you wreak havoc on your immune system. But when you reduce or stop eating sugar, your immune system begins to function correctly. Chronic inflammation is linked to high sugar consumption, which lowers your immune response. When you stop eating sugar, you're likely to find you'll feel better and less likely to catch a cold or bug. One reason for this has to do with your white blood cells. For up to 5 hours after you've eaten a bunch of sugar, those cells are 50 percent less able to fight off bad bacteria. I go through periods where I eat it, then crave it, and I have to stop and break the cycle to get off sugar... and then I feel better again. A "sugar buster" type diet is an excellent way to improve your overall well-being and achieve peak clarity and endurance. It permits the body to calm down the raging inflammation we tend to have. Talk to a dietary specialist or nutritionist to get help for your individual needs.

Another factor to consider is to stop consuming caffeine, alcohol, and other substances. These only mask symptoms and do not help inflammation. I am very sensitive to caffeine. If I drink half of the diet coke at lunchtime, I won't sleep that night. Alcohol makes the pain go away temporarily, but for me in the long run it just exacerbates pain, causes dehydration, and affects my vitamin B levels. When doing any sort of elimination diet, remember to change only one thing at a time, or you won't know what works or doesn't. It can take time to discover the culprit but use your phone, calendar, a journal, or an app to note what you ate and how you felt, which will help make the changes you feel over time more manageable to see. Picking up on patterns is key to figuring out how to help yourself.

The way of eating that helped me

I have found the ketogenic (keto) diet very important in refurbishing my energy levels and renewing my brain function. Ketogenic works with your body to achieve ketosis by eating a low-carb diet (such as the Atkins diet or South Beach diet). The idea is to consume more calories from protein and fat and less from carbohydrates. You cut back most on the carbs that are easy to digest, such as sugar, soda, pastries, and white bread. Ketosis happens when your carbohydrate intake is low, and your body turn to fat as fuel. As your body breaks down fat, it produces an acid called ketones or ketone bodies, which becomes your body and brain's main source of energy. There are numerous benefits of going keto.

I'm in a weight-loss program at the VCU Medical University with Dr. Christine Wolver that uses the ketogenic diet. I have experienced profound changes in my energy levels and cognition abilities on the keto diet, and am able to lose weight. A keto diet also cuts out the carbs and sugar that led to me feeling worse and experiencing heightened inflammation. It is hard to give up the chips and the chocolate, but I always tell myself, "I like feeling better every day, better than how good that might taste for a moment!"

Giving up bread, pasta, sugar, alcohol, chocolate, and bad carbs is not easy. But if you are like me, you will try anything to feel better. One place to start is with the basics of what you put into your body every day. But any changes should be gradual. Don't force yourself to follow strict diets that make you feel stressed out to the point of being counterproductive. Follow the guidance of intuitive eating where you listen to your body.

The most important thing that I can say about what you should do about what you put in your body is to drink more water. Many studies have shown that water intake can improve symptoms allowing an improved blood pressure response to standing in patients with autonomic dysfunctions. Dysautonomia International recommends two liters of water and five grams of salt daily. I carry around a huge 78-ounce water jug I lovingly call the "water woobie." It's also imperative if you have POTS to get plenty of electrolytes and salt. Sports drinks (such as Gatorade Zero with no sugar) hydrate you better than water because the carbs, salt, and other electrolytes help your body absorb fluids. Instead, I take salt tablets (Salt Stick) and drink electrolyte drink mixes (Nuun or Ultimate Replenisher) in my water every day, and it reduces my POTS symptoms by increasing the amount of blood flow.

Please note that many people with EDS can also have small intestinal bacterial overgrowth (SIBO), which can be misdiagnosed as IBS. SIBO can cause issues digesting or metabolizing sucrose and fat, which rules out the keto diet high in fat and protein. Again, please consult with your doctor about what way of eating works best for you.

Minerals and supplements

Ensuring your body has all the proper nutrients is essential, especially when your body is sick and depleted. Many people with EDS are low in essential vitamins, minerals, and nutrients. Many doctors say a good marker to look for is an imbalance in vitamin D. You might also have anemia and low blood iron, which can really affect your energy, as can a low vitamin B. A functional medicine doctor or your general practitioner can run a panel of tests to evaluate whether you are deficient in any particular areas (home tests available online at Everlywell.com).

It's a relatively easy and straightforward fix to adjust your vitamins and minerals. Minerals and supplements are vital to providing nutrients, especially if you have gut issues where you're not correctly absorbing through your intestinal tract. In my case, I had to have several iron infusions initially to get my anemia under control. Now I simply take iron pills to keep my blood strong, and it is no longer an issue.

Many EDSers follow the Cusack protocol for supplementing and eating, and it seems to help some. The Cusack protocol is eight specific nutritional supplements that can reportedly improve connective tissue integrity, and some say it is helpful for mast cell issues.

These are a few essential supplements that have helped me:

- *Magnesium* – I take magnesium (400 mg every night) to help with muscle fatigue. Be aware that magnesium can make you have loose stools, and magnesium citrate can cause a histamine reaction in some people.

- *Calcium* – It helps strengthen my bones so I don't get bone loss, which is expected as we age. I also like Viactiv chocolate calcium chews.

- *Vitamin D* – Many patients with hypermobility are deficient in vitamin D. I initially took 10,000 IUDs every day to replenish my deprived system, but now I only take 500 every few days to ward off a deficiency building back up again.

- *Vitamin B-complex and vitamin C* – These essential supplements help with immunity and well-being. I take 500 mg of each every day. Vitamin B12 needs to be taken regularly because if you stop taking it after eliminating a deficiency, your levels will drop again. Be cautious not to overdo your vitamin B6.

- *Turmeric curcumin* – A wonderful anti-inflammatory supplement that helps with healing when taken regularly.

- *Lion's mane mushroom* – As recommended by my POTS cardiologist, I take lion's mane mushroom in capsule form and drink lion's mane teas to help my cognitive functioning.

- *L-methyl folate* – 15 mg also helps my body absorb nutrients better.

Be sure to see a doctor, whether primary, functional, or gastro, and have your blood levels checked for your potential deficiencies by a professional before taking any supplements. There are some excellent EDS-knowledgeable nutritionists and registered dieticians who can help.

It can also be helpful to try a food sensitivities test to understand what could be causing inflammation or reaction such as the MRT Food Sensitivities Test. A simple food sensitivity blood test can offer tremendous assistance in reducing reactions and inflammation. By getting these foods identified and eliminating them in your diet, you will in turn decrease inflammation in the body that helps to cause your subluxations.

Choose to Assess, Act, or Affirm

- **Assess:** Have you had an evaluation of your urine and/or blood done to see where you might have nutritional deficiencies that supplements could relieve?

- **Act:** Buy a home test such as the EverlyWell Vitamin D and Inflammation Test. The EverlyWell test looks for vitamin D levels and measures C-reactive protein (CRP), which the liver makes when there is inflammation in the body. This finger prick test allows a person to easily collect their blood sample and send it off to a lab for testing. Independent, board-certified doctors will review the results and explain them in easy-to-understand terms. The company then sends the results to a person's online account, which they access via a secure login.

- **Affirm:** "I will focus on being present over perfect."

NOTES

CHAPTER 12

MASSAGE AND PHYSICAL THERAPY

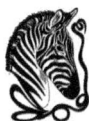

It can be addictive to run yourself ragged. I know. Your heart beats faster, you feel like the thrill of a rush, and your brain feels like it's about to burst with all of your ideas and plans. You're constantly going, going, going, with no stop to it. But chasing that feeling is also damaging your health in the long run. If your head is hurting or you feel tired, take a rest. You're not lazy for needing a break. It's your body's way of telling you that it's been running at full speed for far too long. Listen to your body.

—Melissa Chu

For most people, a headache is just a headache. But for someone with EDS, it can be caused by any one of these many factors:

- Migraines;
- Chiari malformation;
- Cervicogenic headaches;
- Blurry vision;
- POTS / dysautonomia;
- Tethered cord syndrome (TCF);
- Spontaneous cerebro-spinal fluid (CSF) leak;
- Craniocervical instability;
- Temporo-mandibular joint (TMJ) dysfunction;
- Idiopathic intracranial hypertension.

Not such a simple headache anymore, huh? For a passing headache you also probably take aspirin, Tylenol, or Motrin to help ease the pain. But if you're facing chronic pain, doing this for long periods can wreak havoc on your stomach. It's not a healthy long-term solution.

It's essential to find the source of the pain and treat the root cause, which is not always possible. For me, I had to fix my craniocervical instability. However, when we lock down one part of our bodies through fusions or stabilizing braces, other parts can get bent out of shape next. I have progressive spinal stenosis and scoliosis now that my neck is fused, so I try to get myofascial release from massage while improving my strength through physical therapy. One releases while the other strengthens.

Physical therapy (PT)

Physical therapy is an absolute must for people with hypermobile EDS. Loose joints can lead to rigid muscles. Subluxation is the partial dislocation of a joint from its socket, which can cause either a joint to jam and be stuck or loose, both often causing excruciating muscle spasms as the muscles try to hold onto the strained joint. Many people with EDS also will completely dislocate their joints. When your joints and connective tissue move more than they should, logic says you have to strengthen your muscles to hold you upright, increase stability and reduce subluxations. An EDS-knowledgeable PT can help you realign joints and build strength to avoid future subluxations.

Physical therapists have several excellent tools in their toolbox and can teach you how to self-manage your pain at home with tape for joints to reduce strain, bands for stretching and strengthening, and foam rollers to reduce spasms. I have a small home gym of these types of items, and they really help.

One of the critical challenges in hypermobility is called proprioception. This is the sense you have of your joint(s) in space. We have sensors in our bodies that tell our brain where our bodies are in relation to gravity. It senses our joints, tendons, ligaments, muscles, and even skin to send a message to our brain of the exact position of our joints. This helps us walk, use our arms and legs, and maintain our posture without literally tipping over. It is also designed to help protect us from hyperextending our joints and stretching our muscles. When EDS patients have poor proprioception, they cannot tell their joints in relation to their bodies. Many people with hypermobility struggle with poor proprioception in their hands and fingers, and as a result, drop things, sublux, or hold things too tightly. These can all cause pain. Others may face issues with joints hyperextending.

A common symptom for many EDSers (usually tall and thin with long arms and legs) is to have an S-shaped spine—called a "kyphotic curve" in the upper back (bowing forward) and a "lordotic curve" in the lower spine and hips (curving backward). Many people call this a swayback posture. This causes your physical frame to bow in and out from shoulders to knees and puts constraints and pain on your spine and joints.

This physique is a classic sign of hypermobility. It can result in double-jointed knees, sometimes referred to as "banana knees," because they bow backward (hyperextend) farther than they should. At the same time, this slouched posture (due to ligament laxity) often causes ribs to pop out of place. A physical therapist might teach you how to roll on a foam roller under your back to relieve the muscle spasms and get your ribs back into place. Compression garments and orthotic vests/shirts also can be helpful to maintain stability in your core.

I see a PT specialist who focuses on women's pelvic floor issues. She is interviewed in the Appendix of this book. She has helped me learn to stabilize my lower back and core with specific exercises at home to better hold my posture and reduce the pain of frequent subluxations, helping me better manage my "coat hanger pain" that is centralized like a coat hanger sitting on top of my neck and upper shoulders. She believes the pelvic floor is a crucial evaluation for any EDS hypermobile patient to investigate, especially before becoming pregnant.

Physical therapy also can help with flat feet and gait. EDSers have unstable ankles, which can lead to unsteady legs, knees, hips, and spine. Many people can curve their ankles around, walk on the edges of their feet, or roll their ankles while walking. This can cause pain in the side of the lower leg. Improving a person's gait can correct how they walk, which helps reduce instability and pain in the rest of the body. Some people swear by shoe inserts or orthotics that stabilize the feet. A podiatrist can help determine what's best for your feet.

No matter what your issue is, when you engage in regular therapy with a PT, you need to understand that you will not be like others near you receiving treatment. They will be steadily and even rapidly progressing and getting stronger, better, and back to normal after an injury. For EDSers the key is to start very low and go slow (think turtle pace). If you push yourself excessively, you may cause damage to your fragile tissue that takes longer to heal. Do not do too much in one day.

It is difficult to accept, but you need to understand that if you have hypermobility you may be a lifelong physical

HOLD YOUR HEAD UP MUCH?

Do you frequently hold your chin or head up with your hand on the elbow? It's a common symptom of neck instability. Hypermobile EDS is about fragile connective tissue and often comes with loose or lax ligaments like elastic bands. Your muscles are working overtime just to hold up your bowling ball-weighted head.

Try wearing a rigid neck collar most of the day for a few weeks to see if you get pain relief. Wearing a brace can reduce the pain and the frequent subluxation of the joints common in hEDS. When subluxation happens in your neck, you can have what's called cranial settling—where the skull presses on the lower part of the brain, causing pressure, swelling, and a lot of neurological issues. It can push the brain through the hole in the bottom of your skull, sometimes creating real or false Chiari malformation.

I suggest either the Vista Aspen Multipost collar (available on Amazon) or the Miami J collar depending on whether you have TMJ. (You can get it custom fitted at an orthotic center such as Hanger Clinics.) Both are used to stabilize the weak ligaments and muscles to hold up your head.

therapy patient. You will progress, regress, progress again, and the cycle of maintaining your best wellness is the best you can and will achieve if you do the work. This is the mindset you need to have to succeed in PT with EDS: You are working as best you can with what you have. You must do your home exercises as set by your PT to optimize the strength in your muscles to counterbalance your laxity issues. If you regularly do your PT, as painful as it can be, you will feel better in the long run than when you are not doing it. I know it's easier said than done, but when you put in the effort to take these measures to better care for yourself, you will find significant improvements in your pain levels.

Massage

As I could afford it, I would indulge infrequently on vacations, self-care days, and later in life for chronic pain. I feel at my best when I can afford to get a therapeutic massage about once every 6–8 weeks. Find a great provider (medical massage therapists are covered by some insurance), and see them regularly as you can. But be sure to find someone versed in EDS or willing to learn – **to a hypermobile person, there *is* such a thing as a bad massage.**

If you cannot locate or afford massage at any regular interval, find alternative care techniques. Stretching in water is beneficial for pain. Gentle yoga and mindful movement can help with strength building and stress relief. There are so many resources on YouTube that you can find a guided visualization or something to ease your spasmed muscles just a bit. Be creative in thinking about teaching your brain to tell your body to relax. Build the relaxation skill.

One increasingly popular option is dry needling, where a tiny needle penetrates the skin to treat underlying muscular trigger points for the management of neuromusculoskeletal pain. When dry needling is applied to a dysfunctional muscle or trigger point, it can decrease muscle tightness, increase blood flow, and reduce both local and referred pain. I have seen the benefits myself although it can be painful in the short term, but it provides a longer-lasting muscle relaxant benefit. Learn more before you try it. It's not suitable for everyone.

Find creative ways to achieve homeostasis. If you have a physical therapist, physiatrist, or other rehabilitation practitioners, please remember to check with them first before starting a new routine.

Choose to Assess, Act, or Affirm

- **Assess:** What forms of physiotherapy or other manual release methods do you benefit from? Are there any new ones you would like to try next?

- **Act:** Read about "acupressure for beginners." It will give you a good understanding of acupressure pressure points from many perspectives, including how they are used, how to find them, and how to press them. You'll also find information on acupressure point names and guidelines. It's a simple, easy, and free way to open up health and healing. It literally puts the power to help yourself and others in your own hands.

- **Affirm:** "I will remain a profound, powerful soul for the remainder of my life."

Bibliography

Acupressure Points. Acupressure for Beginners. (n.d.). https://acupressure.com/acupressure-basics/acupressure-points/.

NOTES

PART V

HEALING HABITS FOR YOUR SOUL

In this final part I focus attention on the aspects of a medical condition that I believe do not get enough attention in most hypermobile books and resources—your heart and soul. This is where we all need support—in making a connection. There are plenty of books with medical information and resources galore to overwhelm your mind with facts, data, and prognoses. But I feel it is important to also discuss the emotional or spiritual side. It needs healing too.

In this section, I remind you that self-care is not selfish and share tips on how to prioritize your needs when you need it most. I place attention on the nature of how your relationships with family, friends, partners, and co-workers can change during illness, my theories on why this happens, and how to keep your team supportive. Finally there are several listings and links to useful medical resources, support groups, and thousands of hours of online reference material to deepen your research, including a few key hEDS patient groups who globally support zebras and their unique challenges. Healing is not a solo act, and we all need a little help from time to time.

CHAPTER 13

MAKE TIME FOR SELF-CARE

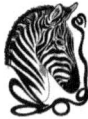

When we neglect ourselves, we deprive ourselves of what we need: attention, consideration, care, support, reassurance, connection, encouragement, and love. We then tend to look toward others to provide it for us. We mistakenly believe that the pain we experience is something only they can soothe or heal. I guess that's why we don't do it for ourselves. The problem is that others cannot do it for us. They cannot fill the void we create depriving ourselves of self-care.

—Marlena Tillhon

Making time for self-care is one of the most important —and hardest—lessons to learn. This chapter could probably go at the beginning of this book as it is so critical that it is tough to do the other habits without it.

People often tell me they don't know what self-care is. They are used to living in a chronic state of being overwhelmed and fatigued, disregarding their own needs to take care of others. They intellectually realize neither "fighting" nor "fleeing" is sustainable but often don't do anything about it.

We often hear that our brains are hard-wired for fight-or-flight and that "we evolved this way," but we know now that our brains can be rewired. It can be challenging, even under the best of circumstances, to find the time to exercise, choose to cook and eat healthy foods, and get enough rest. I do not minimize the daily challenge.

It's far more difficult when you're struggling with the melancholy of challenges that also accompany chronic illness. One day can be good, and one day you can't. But taking good care of yourself is vital for your physical and mental well-being when addressing chronic illness. It brings an added benefit—practicing healthy habits can help you feel that you're regaining control of your life again.

Self-care is the practice of taking an active role in protecting your own well-being and having the ability, tools, and resources to respond to periods of stress so that they don't result in imbalance. **Self-care means asking yourself what you need and following through with an honest answer.** It can be as simple as going to bed earlier or as hard as taking a hard look at some of the habits you've created for yourself.

Why self-care matters

Doing kind, compassionate, and caring things for ourselves, particularly when we are struggling, can help us cope and move through difficult emotional experiences. Countless research findings demonstrate the importance of one's ability to attend to and meet personal needs. For instance, self-care has increased empathy and immunologic functioning and decreased anxiety and depression.

Self-care activities can be sensory, emotional, physical, spiritual, and social. The idea of initiating self-care and integrating it into everyday life is to find out what feels good to you—something that you genuinely enjoy doing and that fits your lifestyle and your values. Self-care is often confused with self-indulgence or anything enjoyable, but it is not a justification for doing what feels good. Authentic self-care will recharge your batteries. For example, while drinking a glass or two of wine certainly might feel good, you know it's not good for you, and it's not going to help you restore your emotional or physical well-being.

Self-care can also seem selfish when you are accustomed to helping other people, as many women do regularly. However, it allows people to take better care of others because self-care ensures that we have taken care of our needs, so we operate from a state of inner balance, which renders us better equipped to meet others' needs. This is particularly hard for those of us (myself included) who struggle with patience. We have to take on the challenge of being a kind and patient friend to ourselves and make the time to figure out what brings us joy and how to make time for that.

While self-care may sound simple enough, it is often challenging to execute. One of the most common reasons for people not engaging in regular self-care is that they "don't have time." Fortunately, you can do many different self-care practices, none of which are incredibly time-consuming or require a lot of money or planning. Once self-care becomes a part of everyday life, you will likely become more and more protective of that time and wonder how you ever managed without it.

CAMILLE SCHRIER, MISS AMERICA 2020 ON THE IMPORTANCE OF SELF-CARE

"It feels selfish sometimes. Honestly, even when I'm not able to see people that I want to see because I'm too tired to get together to socialize, or I have to say no to things because of EDS, even though I want to go because I know that I need to rest. Or when I need to go and go to the doctor or go to the grocery store to make sure that I have food to eat through the week so I'm not scrambling. There are so many things that I have to do to prevent a lot of the flares and symptoms and it takes me away from a lot of the things that I might like to do. But I also have to just tell myself I can do that when I feel better or when I have energy to do it. We need self-care. It's important."

How to practice self-care

Are you the type of person who's too busy driving from place to place to stop and fill that gas tank with the beaming low fuel light? Too busy rushing about to take a moment? Too guilty to take a pause even though it's clear you need one? Perhaps, you don't feel empowered enough to demand a break? Or maybe you're just so caught up in your day that it's easier to ignore all the signs telling you it's time to pause, breathe, and assess the situation. The warning light is on, but we often ignore it and keep on driving until it becomes a bigger problem.

We can evolve beyond fight-or-flight responses by moving toward two new responses—empathy and action—both of which start with self-care. **The most courageous self-care act is learning to say, "I need help."**

Identifying the need for a "personal moment" of self-care is critical. Where we tend to fall short is acting on our own recognition. It's not enough just to notice that low fuel light inside your head. You have to do what it's telling you—pull over, put it in park, and refuel. This isn't always easy and, in fact, often requires a good bit of personal courage.

1. *The Pre-Ask: Asking for Help or Space Before You Actually Need It*

   Most people refuse to ask for help or acknowledge that they need a little space until their anxiety is already at a boiling point. Let's go back to the "low fuel" light analogy. When the light comes on, you know you've only got about 30 miles before running out of gas. But, hey, that's still 30 miles! No need to start looking for a gas station immediately. Why worry about what's going to happen down the road, right? In the case of self-care, it's the accumulation of stressors that haven't been addressed that switch on that light. These stressors get more and more critical as you head down life's road, piling up and piling on until you find yourself with an empty tank—or burnout. In other words, don't wait too long. You will get exhausted from simple things and feel super frustrated by that. Let those you trust know when you feel like you're approaching the point of needing help or a step back. Give them time to prepare themselves to be more effective when you do reach out.

2. *The Kindness Factor: Remember That People Love to Help*

Think about the last time you helped someone or were willing to recognize their need for space. Chances are you came out of the experience feeling a powerful sense of gratification, goodwill, and pride. That's because we humans love helping each other. We're hard-wired for empathy. We like doing good things for one another, which is why acts of kindness, large and small, happen worldwide every day. Therefore, it stands to reason that there are plenty of people in your life who at one time or another would have been happy to help you had they been asked. They would have gladly watched your kids, assisted with the project on which you were stuck, or just given you the space you needed to take a moment of reflection. The problem was usually not their willingness to help you. The problem was and is your fear and inability to reach out with the ask.

People who want to help are out there. But you have to open the door and invite them inside.

And one of the most important things you can do besides asking for help is preparing to ask for help. A self-care plan is a fail-safe created by you and filled with your favorite self-care activities, important reminders, and ways to activate your self-care community. Here's why it's crucial to create your own self-care plan:

1. *Customizing a self-care plan is a preventative measure.* By designing a navigational road map that is unique to you, in moments when you're *not* in crisis, you're directing your best self to reflect on what you may need (and have access to) in your worst moments. The reality is that only *you* know how intense your stress levels can get and what resources are available to you.

2. *Having a plan takes the guesswork out of what to do and where to turn in moments of crisis.* From a mindfulness point of view, it helps you respond instead of reacting to the situation at hand. You'll feel more in control of your circumstances when you have a plan in place, and life won't feel quite as chaotic. (It also makes it easier to ask for help from those with whom you share your plan.)

3. *A self-care plan helps you stay the course.* You'll find it far easier to stick to your personal care strategy and avoid falling into the trap of making excuses or not prioritizing yourself first. A plan helps you establish a routine, ensuring that you and your self-care partners don't wind up in isolation. You can check in with each other, hold each other accountable, and share the responsibility to support one another.

Ideas for self-care

There are hundreds of ways that you can take care of yourself. Some people think self-care is about getting a massage or getting your nails done. Those are helpful, but self-care is so much simpler. You could cross off something on your to-do list, not do it today, and do it when you feel up to it. It can be as easy as having a glass of lemonade. One of my favorite things to do for self-care is going to Chick-fil-A and getting a diet lemonade. It makes me so happy. What simple thing makes you so happy? Go do it!

I recommend you make a list of your top 10 things that you do for self-care and prioritize when you can do them daily, weekly, monthly, or as needed—and start practicing forcing those things into your schedule by waking up every morning and thinking about what you can do to squeeze a little bit of joy into today. Find opportunities to use your strengths—the things that energize you. Examples of self-care you can do today are literally too numerous to count, but here's a short list to consider:

Emotional self-care

- Learn to say no.
- Intentionally schedule "me time" on your calendar or planner.
- Reward yourself for completing small tasks.
- Use online tutorials to learn something new.
- Allow yourself to feel and express your feelings (in a safe and appropriate environment).
- Try some adult coloring as a form of anxiety and/or stress release.
- Stop being your harshest critic. Allow yourself to make mistakes.

Physical self-care

- Take a walk.
- Go for a car ride to nowhere in particular.
- Go spend some time in nature.
- Go to bed early.

Social self-care

- Choose who you spend your time with today. Spend time with people who are enthusiastic and positive.

- Join a support group for people going through what you're going through.

- Schedule a regular date night with your significant other.

Sleep as self-care

Routinely sleeping six or fewer hours a night can wreak havoc on your immune system, double your cancer risk, and cause anxiety and depression. Despite the health risks, many of us don't take sleep seriously, choosing instead to sacrifice it in favor of things like working, socializing, scrolling social media, and playing video games. Learn and focus seriously on prioritizing sleep. It will return rewards in spades.

For me, self-care is about rest and sleep. When I am relaxed, my muscles are finally at ease from the constant state of contraction needed to literally hold my bones and joints together. You need to rest a lot if you're chronically ill—sometimes you're frustrated by how much you need to rest, but ultimately it is good for you and is a healing thing.

According to a fall 2020 survey from the American Academy of Sleep Medicine (AASM), roughly one-third of Americans reported difficulties with sleep. The struggle for a good night's sleep has led to an increase in sleep aids. According to the AASM survey, 51 percent of those surveyed reported using medication, over-the-counter supplements, or other substances to help them fall asleep. But rather than turn to medicine, try implementing some of the tips the AASM recommends to promote high-quality sleep:

1. *Keep a schedule.* If you want to wake up at 7:00 a.m., plan to head for the bedroom around 10:00 p.m. the night before. Avoid staying up and sleeping later on the weekends, and limit naps to early in the afternoon and roughly 20 to 30 minutes. Set a bedtime that is early enough for you to get at least seven hours of sleep.

2. *Ditch the screens.* At least 30 minutes before bedtime, turn off or put away any electronic devices. Lose the blue light and the addiction of having the phone in your hand and checking your social media accounts. Don't go to bed unless you're sleepy.

3. *Stay active.* Exercise regularly but not right before bedtime.

4. *Don't fret.* If you're having difficulty dropping off, doctors recommend a warm bath, listening to music, or winding down through meditation or prayer. Avoid consuming caffeine in the late afternoon or evening.

5. *Do fret.* For those whose minds just won't settle, Dr. Samuel A. Taylor recommends setting a "worry hour" when it suits you. Worry about everything very hard for 60 minutes, and then allow yourself to stop and enjoy the rest of your day.

Make the investment

"Ask yourself if you're living your life in the most meaningful way. What would you prefer not to do? Who would you want to spend more time with? You will never get more time in your life, so start to make changes now."

—Olessia Kantor

There are countless therapies, apps, and tools out there that you can try to relieve your pain, ease your fatigue, and sleep better or whatever symptom with which you are trying to resolve. Many are not covered by health insurance. Below I share a few basic recommendations and insights I have learned over the years. I recommend these things be a regular part of your self-care routine. Consult your care provider(s) before beginning any of these suggestions based on your individual needs. Included is an ongoing list of products I have tried, used, and ones that failed. As soon as this book is printed, it will be out-of-date. I maintain an updated list on the book's website at www. holdingitalltogether.com for the latest version. Note: No affiliation with any of the products or services listed.

These suggestions may cost you time and/or money. Research and invest in things that may work for you. Everyone's experience will be different, so I pass these on to you as a potential resource. Maybe you'll experience a positive snowball effect, with good results and benefits rolling and cascading into an avalanche of healing.

- *The Fascia Blaster:* A patented muscle tool to help relax chronically tightened muscles. I find it very helpful to relieve spasms. There are different sizes with various types of claws to penetrate different muscle groups. Amazon says it is "the #1 selling self-massage myofascial tool for massaging your tissue." It touts the benefits of temporarily increasing blood flow to the working areas of your body. Amazon also says, "Added bonus, the FasciaBlaster temporarily lessens the appearance of cellulite." I just know it releases extremely tight muscle spasms.

- *The Body Braid:* This unique body wrapping tool helps me pull joints and muscles gently into proper position. I use it on my shoulders to pull them back into alignment with my spine and head. Check it out online at www.thebodybraid.com.

- *Bongers:* Acupressure tools that you bang on trigger points to release spastic muscles as needed. It can also bring circulation to the part of your extremities you focus on banging gently or as an acupressure point for additional potential pain relief.

- *BodyBackBuddy tool:* This S-shaped muscle relaxation "digging" tool is suitable for spasms you cannot reach, for example, on your back.

- *Dynamic Cupping:* My masseuse uses these soft silicon cupping sets of various sizes to aid in circulation to tight muscle spasms regularly bound up in my shoulders and back. I got a set for home for less than $20 and my PT taught me how to use them. I find it very effective if you can handle the short-term pain and the bruising it causes.

- *TheraBands:* For affordable home rubber resistance bands for dynamic stretching and gentle strength building.

- *Foam Rollers:* For the occasions you need to roll out a painful subluxed joint back into place. Get your PT to help teach you how.

- *TheraICE Headache & Migraine Relief Hat:* Can reduce inflammation and reduce tension or stress-related headaches.

- *Dr Teal's Epsom Salts*: A cup or two added to your warm bath for soaking is a cheap and easy way to soothe sore muscles, aid in recovery, and pain relief.

- *Compression clothes:* I find that compression shirts or tank tops that primarily cover my torso are the most helpful. I tried compression socks at my cardiologist's advice and on many public forums. It helped me with the blood that pooled in my feet and ankles, but they're not very comfortable to wear all day or every day. I have seen several posts recommending wearing thigh-high stockings as compression wear. They are available on several sites online and in stores.

- *Magsoothium:* A magnesium and arnica blend soothing pain cream. Available on their website and on Amazon in varieties of cooling, warming, and with CDB.

- *Salt Stick Fast Chews:* Maintaining healthier than average levels of salts helps the fluidity of our blood flow. Orange is my favorite flavor.

- *Electrolyte drink mixes:* If you have POTS, it is helpful to get enough fluid in to enhance your blood circulation. I like Nuun tablets and Ultimate Replenisher 1–2 times a day in my water. In addition, occasionally I need to increase my magnesium when feeling extra fatigued or sensitive to barometric weather changes. Then I also add products such as LYTEshow, Liquid IV, or Natural Vitality Calm magnesium powder in my water.

- *CBD products:* There are many sources and not agreed-upon standards, so buyer beware. I use a home farm supplier where I can order online at www.804hemp.com.

- *Prism glasses:* These are important to avoid cervical spine overuse, particularly with craniocervical instability. They have a mirror to allow you to look down without bending your neck forward.

- *Pulse oximeter:* Get this low-tech home device to learn the patterns of your heart rate and blood oxygenation. Learn what activities increase and decrease your heart rate or cause palpitations.

- *HRV monitor:* Heart rate variability (HRV) can increase vagal tone and improve tachycardia with POTS. I like these two products to be used in order. First, get a 4–8 week subscription to a Lief Therapeutics heart monitor device and app for becoming more aware of your HRV. Once you are more aware, get an Oura ring to train to recover and enhance your HRV.

In addition to the products above are my favorite self-management apps to check out:

- **Calm** (https://www.calm.com/): In my opinion the best, easiest way to learn mindful breathing to calm the nervous system and foster healing.

- **3 Good Things** (https://the3goodthings.org/about): A simple gratitude tracker for daily journaling.

- **Medisafe** (https://www.medisafeapp.com/): A simple medication management tool with reminder for seamless management of tracking what you take and when.

- **Curable** (https://www.curablehealth.com/): Training on the brain-pain relationship to reduce pain suffering.

- **My ID** (https://shop.getmyid.com/): Great basic medical app to keep on your smartphone. It allows you to store all your relevant medical information, including your conditions, medications, insurance information, which can be shared with first aid responders.

- **Pip Stress Tracker** (https://thepip.com/): Personal stress management tracking device.

- **Fooducate** (https://www.fooducate.com/): An app community for healthy eating, tracking calories, and more.

- **Gratitude** (https://gratefulness.me/): A simple app that allows you to document something that you're grateful for every day. It's useful if you're not interested in writing out journal entries and prefer to diarize random thoughts.

- **MyFitnessPal** (https://www.myfitnesspal.com/): A simple app journal for weight tracking, food, exercise, and daily water consumption.

- **Endive** (https://endive.app/): An app that allows you to document and track each meal you eat and any gut health-related symptoms for IBS and more. It helps monitor triggers you pick up on and then is compiled into a weekly report for you to look back over to review and analyze patterns.

- **Cozi** (https://www.cozi.com/): A calendaring app to use with your family to help you manage your multiple schedules.

- **Flaredown** (http://flaredown.com/): A trigger tracking app where you check in daily to give a brief update on your conditions, symptoms, treatments, the health factors that have affected you, and to give a final summary of that day so you can pick up on trends.

- **Youper** (https://www.youper.ai/): An option for mental health support with or without insurance that can monitor and improve your emotional health via talks based on therapy techniques or mindfulness.

- **Pathways** (https://www.pathways.health/): An app that you can use to help you manage your pain through guided meditation, visualization, sound, and more.

- **Manage My Pain (MMP)** (https://managemypainapp.com/): A great app if you suffer from any form of chronic pain; it can be used to document and report on its severity.

- **Lauren's Hope** (http://www.laurenshope.com): Fashionable medical identification jewelry.

- **Stop, Breath & Think** (https://stopbreathethink.com/): Recommends activities paired with your current emotions, no matter if you're anxious, hopeful, angry, or just can't fall asleep.

- **Rootd** (https://www.rootd.io/): A mental health app meant for people who suffer from debilitating panic attacks and anxiety with a featured self-help "panic button" to ease panic attacks.

- **Day One** (https://dayoneapp.com/): A journaling app that gives you a clear and easy way to document anything you'd like to keep tabs on including voice notes, photos, or even videos along with the text.

- **MyLinks** (https://www.mylinks.com/): A free application to help you gather, manage, and share all of your personal health records from one secure location, fully under your control.

- **Mindshift** (www.anxietycanda.com): Free cognitive behavioral therapy strategies to try.

- **Clear Free** (https://www.clearfear.co.uk/): Free anxiety coping skills.

- **SuperBetter** (https://www.superbetter.com/): Free resources to build resilience, achieve goals, and tackle challenges.

- **WhatsUp:** (https://www.thewhatsupapp.co.uk/): Free strategies to manage anxiety, anger, depression, stress, and low self-esteem.

Choose to Assess, Act, or Affirm

- **Assess:** Be honest with yourself: Do you actively practice some form of self-care on most days?
- **Act:** Remind yourself that you've got this. You are capable and can handle anything that comes your way.
- **Affirm:** "I trust myself and the process of achieving my aspirations."

Bibliography

American Academy of Sleep Medicine. (2021). "Americans continue struggling for a good night's sleep during the pandemic." https://aasm.org/americans-struggling-good-nights-sleep-during-pandemic/.

"A Guide to Practicing Self-Care with Mindfulness." (n.d.). Mindful.org. https://www.mindful.org/a-guide-to-practicing-self-care-with-mindfulness/.

Mills, J., Wand, T., & Fraser, J.A. (2015). "On Self-Compassion and Self-Care in Nursing: Selfish or Essential for Compassionate Care?" *Int J Nurs Stud*, 52(4): 791–793. doi: 10.1016/j.ijnurstu.2014.10.009.

"Self care vision board." (n.d.). PositivePsychology.com. https://positivepsychology.com/wp-content/uploads/Self-Care-Vision-Board.pdf

Schure, M.B., Christopher, J.C., and Christopher, S. (2008). "Mind-Body Medicine and the Art of Self-Care: Teaching Mindfulness to Counseling Students through Yoga, Meditation, and Qigong." *Journal of counseling and development*, 86(1). doi:10.1002/j.1556–6678.2008.tb00625.x

Tygielski, S., and Rossy, L. (2018). "Self-Care Is an Act of Resistance." Mindful.org. https://www.mindful.org/self-care-is-an-act-of-resistance/.

NOTES

CHAPTER 14

MAINTAINING RELATIONSHIPS

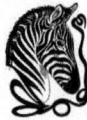

Butterflies have a liquid in the core of their body, and as they struggle to get out of the cocoon, that liquid is pushed into the veins in the butterfly wings where it hardens and makes the wings strong. If the butterfly doesn't push and pull and fight to get out of the cocoon, its wings won't be strong enough to fly, and the butterfly dies. Without the struggle, there are no wings. Do not take away someone's opportunity to grow by trying to "fix" them or rescue them from their trials. Without the struggle, they would not have their wings.

—Lora Devries

I t is difficult to acknowledge and admit, but often our relationships can suffer when we are chronically ill. It is natural to withdraw when we are stressed. Perhaps we all evolved to withdraw when alarmed as a survival strategy, as when early humans encountered predators and hiding helped save them. Nor does everyone understand what you are dealing with or wants to ride along to the depths of despair you can allow yourself to venture into or the hopelessness you sometimes feel.

It's sad, but even the people closest to us often dismiss or disbelieve that your invisible illness even exists. Lack of support is one of the most difficult things when you're lost in a new diagnosis and challenges finding help or treatment. It hurts deeply when loved ones don't have your back. Unfortunately, this topic comes up a lot more in EDS support groups than it should. This was the case in my family. I know my daughter had a tough time watching her mom decay. After I couldn't work, we had to move from our home for the benefit of a cheaper cost of living, and she must have felt very alone.

The need to disconnect and heal damaged my relationships. I believe this is because so many of us allow ourselves to identify as a "sick person" following a health crisis. It is hard to see yourself as anything else. It has taken me a few years, but I no longer identify as the victimized, woe-is-me persona. I think it is key not accepting the philosophy of being okay with being sick. When you can rise above, others will often follow along. I am just starting to see the fruits of that labor in my family relationships many years later.

It is imperative to maintain the relationships you can as circumstances allow. These relationships can be an invaluable source of practical and emotional support, but it can be difficult for your loved ones to accept your condition, and misunderstandings can easily happen. Many symptoms of hypermobility are invisible, so others cannot always see how we are affected. This makes it hard for them to realize how you are feeling. Knowing when to help can also be difficult for family and friends as it can be hard to know when help will be graciously accepted or when it might feel like interference. Children often find it challenging to see parents in pain or less capable than before. Reassure them and answer any questions they might have and explain you cannot do things the same way as you have in the past. Talk to your closest loved ones about your symptoms and how they affect your daily life, and come up with ideas on how they can help to make life easier for you and for them. You can work through many of these hardships together reminding them you are the same person, just with different needs than before.

When you can no longer get understanding or compassion from your family, it is helpful to turn to friends or other zebras. It is often said that you are born into your family, but you choose your friends. Your friends are special because you have found something in each other worth getting to know and have decided to cultivate that as a bond. Put in the effort, and don't neglect your friends during the busy times. Share memorable moments, and don't let insignificant issues break your friendship.

Many of us spend a lot of time at work (if we are able to work) and may even see our work colleagues as much as our partner. For this reason, a good relationship with work colleagues can make a massive difference in how much you enjoy your job. The relationships you have

I UNDERSTAND LOVED ONES DON'T ALWAYS KNOW HOW TO RESPOND

I have unfortunately been estranged from my family of origin for the past several years following my diagnosis and focus on my health issues. They literally couldn't hear about my issues anymore. I understand that they saw me as negative and a complainer. I am not making excuses, but dealing with chronic pain, subluxations, and weird randomly occurring symptoms can make you feel negative all the time. Together they decided that my mother should "have a talk with me" to request I stop talking about my health.

I knew then I had to make the difficult choice to distance myself from them as a matter of well-being. As of today, I remain at an arm's distance. But it allows me to heal from the family system that doesn't support me like I need to be supported.

I have worked diligently to repair that negative thinking and to retrain my brain. Now I am more educated and know better how to better cope.

The most important thing as any therapist would tell you to do is to gain control of your *reactions* to other people. If you react to stress or get caught up in negativity, your angry response can further alienate people from your life in your time of need. I was resentful and mean to the people closest to me who couldn't help me as I cascaded down. I deeply regret that. We need to accept caregivers for who they are, and most importantly, realize what they can or can't give you. People can only give what they can. Be empathetic to their situation as it is hard to watch someone you care about lose their total capacity to chronic illness such as EDS. Some people with chronic illness can be in denial and never share their symptoms, even though sharing might help them and others. It is especially hard if those around you are also in denial. I have written a short e-book, *Dear Loved One*, to help people with chronic illnesses teach their loved ones how to better communicate with them. You can download it at: https://bit.ly/What-to-say-to-the-chronically-ill.

with others at your place of employment can be tricky if you are still able to work. If you want to maximize your productivity at work, you must learn to make the most of your relationships with your work colleagues. Be on friendly terms with everyone you can. Offer to help, and accept help when offered. Spend lunch or break time together with colleagues, and don't neglect to build relationships outside of work.

No matter your relationship with your parents, it will remain one of the most influential relationships you are a part of throughout your life. Parents can drive us crazy and piss us off, but they are often the ones we turn to when we are looking for support in tough times, understanding family history, or finding the missing pieces of ourselves. Whether your relationship with your parents leans toward positive or negative, there are ways you can enhance the relationship. Show them respect, and learn from their wisdom. Build the connection between them and your children, and ask them about their history. Most of all, make time for each other.

Finally, good relationships with a partner don't just happen. They take work. If you have had a significant other for any amount of time, you know that it takes effort. To make the most of your relationship with your partner, give them priority, have fun together, and learn with them. Regularly express your appreciation, and be creative in showing your love.

Relationships of all kinds are important. That said, it's still essential for you to maintain your individuality; don't allow anyone to mistreat you or disrespect your boundaries. If you are a mom or a caregiver, it is very difficult to put yourself first, but you must come first when you are sick.

Establishing your wellness needs and boundaries

It is vital to figure out your no-go rules or boundaries within your relationships when you become chronically ill. You will change your plans, or skip family dinners and gatherings or events when you don't feel up to it. **You are not required to participate if you have a bad day. You are allowed to have bad days, and self-care is essential.** This can hurt feelings, spoil plans, and negatively affect the other people in your life. Believe me, I understand how hard it is to put yourself first and take care of your own well-being as your number one priority, but it is the best way for you to focus on being well. Remember the old flight attendant routine of why your mask should go on first: You cannot help others if you don't help yourself first.

Once you have determined your boundaries, whatever they may be, stick to them and don't waffle. Make sure that you clearly communicate to others what you expect of them and the consequences of crossing your boundaries. If people cross them, then consider having as minimal contact with them as possible. This is not to be cruel or for attention. It is so you can focus primarily on getting better without distraction, guilt, or blame games.

Having a solid support system and a plan for bad days is vital. Avoid stressful situations as much as possible, including people who stress you out, and allow yourself time to recover from those situations. Don't feel bad asking for help—it is what you need and does not mean you are weak. Living with hypermobility can be emotionally as well as physically challenging. Some people may find their mobility and independence affected, which can also change the way they live, the way they see themselves or relate to others. You may feel misunderstood, guilty, or worry you are not coping as well as you think you should be. But stress, anxiety, and depression are not "all in your head" and neither is chronic illness. They are a very real part of the common challenges and can become more severe resulting in a negative impact on your ability to manage your condition and your life in general.

Symptoms of anxiety and depression are often not *the* diagnosis but symptoms of the other things you face. The array of difficulties that we deal with often and understandably leads to anxiety and depression, and that's nothing to be ashamed of. I strongly suggest you create your own toolbox, such as videos, music, poems, images, and meditations, that makes you feel calm and peaceful. This could be going to a place that helps or visualizing a calming, happy memory, as well as taking the effort to reach out to friends who can lift you up. When you feel vulnerable, try journaling your feelings to get them out of your system. A diary can be therapeutic and cathartic. Sometimes writing things down can help us feel less overwhelmed and can help us better see any barriers between us and accepting the help we might need. Having an informed, compassionate therapist is critical as well. There is a lot of stuff to work through, and only you can do it alone. There are tons of books on this topic to learn from.

Dealing with toxic relationships when you're not at your best

Suppose you have family or significant others who don't believe that you're actually sick, or they won't take you seriously or listen to you. In that case, ask if they will go to your doctor's appointment(s) and have the doctor explain things to them. Sometimes it takes an outside influence to open people up. You may have a friend that can speak to them on your behalf. Support is critical to your ongoing wellness, so get it where you can—support groups, family, friends, colleagues, or any place with a sympathetic ear. We've all been through some form of struggle. Also, realize that some people may come around in their own time, while others cannot change their ways. That is not your problem. It is theirs. Let them handle it. You have enough on your plate.

Many times a challenge can be other people's toxic positivity. This is when someone says or believes that everything is great, that there are no problems worth discussing, has no issues, and continues to say things will get better regardless. This is also a form of denial, and some people cannot cope with the new you. Others think maybe if we don't talk about it, it will go away. Or my favorite one, "Put that worry in a box inside your mind, seal it up, and forget about it"—as if we don't know the destruction burying our emotions can do to us.

Toxic relationships can be difficult to end, but sometimes, all it takes is knowing the ways they can harm you to convince you to cut ties. There are typically four ways a toxic relationship can harm someone:

1. *Your flight-or-fight response is constantly on:* Have your friends noticed you are more irritable than usual lately? Maybe you seem to get mad at the slightest remark? Being in a toxic relationship keeps your body in a high-stress mode. When you sense anything that could be a threat, you will immediately try to fight it or run away from it. It will leave you feeling run down and empty and leave your friends feeling attacked too.

2. *You'll have physical aches and pains:* The flight-or-fight response results from cortisol, the stress hormone coursing through your veins. When this is in your blood all the time, it can cause all sorts of aches and pains. Think of toxic relationships much like toxic chemicals—they do your body harm and should be avoided like poison!

3. *You will lose sleep:* Besides just cortisol, if you are constantly fighting with, or fearful of, a toxic relationship, this can also change other hormones in your body such as adrenaline. When these hormones trigger at the wrong time, this can cause you to have problems, for instance, not sleeping at night. You are never yourself when you don't get enough sleep no matter who you are!

4. *You will lower your self-esteem:* Above all else, a toxic relationship is self-perpetuating. When you constantly feel physical pain and aren't sleeping enough, you will likely feel terrible about yourself. It will

eventually erode your self-esteem. This means more stress, more aches and pains, and the cycle continues.

As difficult as it is, you should consider cutting off truly toxic relationships because of the vast implications for your health and happiness. When you are in that form of a relationship, you will likely feel uncomfortable or even anxious, which can impede healing. You might even be afraid to ask them to do things or not expect them to help you when you need it most. When this happens day in and day out, you will soon think that everyone in the world is like this when they are not. You can become resentful, which is not helpful to you or anyone else. It can foster a pessimistic and unhealthy attitude.

Choose to Assess, Act, or Affirm

- **Assess:** Do you have toxic or unhealthy relationships that leave you drained and feeling unwell?
- **Act:** Take inventory of the people who are there for you when you are at your worst, and stand close to them.
- **Affirm:** "I choose thoughts that create a healthy atmosphere within and around me."

Bibliography

Morris, T. (n.d.). *6 Ways to Add Laughter to Your Life*. Reinvent Yourself. https://teressamorris.com/6-ways-to-add-laughter-to-your-life/.

NOTES

CHAPTER 15

MUSTERING UP SUPPORT

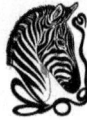

Without a doubt, the most important thing to remember is that it's okay to feel overwhelmed and stressed out. It's okay to feel lost and unsure. It's alright to have no idea how you're going to hold it together sometimes. We put so much pressure on ourselves to be happy all the time. It's okay to acknowledge when times are tough. It's alright to feel anxious, even if it's uncomfortable.

—Ilene S. Cohen

There are many resources you can rely on for support if you have hypermobile EDS. Many people work very hard to advocate for themselves and for others. I have never seen people help others in a community like those in the

EDS community. I have received so much care and advice from a handful of complete strangers who willingly show me such compassion and kindness. It is a gift. There are also many advocacy groups, support groups, and nonprofit organizations where you can find information on EDS—everything from coping skills to just places to find someone who "gets it" when no one else seems to understand.

Advocacy and support groups

When we face any conflict in life, advocacy and support groups can help introduce us to others who are in the same situation as we find ourselves, allowing empathy and understanding on a deeper level. It is often just validating to talk to someone else who might relate to the weird things that our bodies are doing! Those people help me cope and see the sometimes elusive light of hope at the end of a dark tunnel. And on occasion I am able to show them the light too.

Individuals and families affected by rare medical conditions might look to nonprofit support and advocacy groups for different reasons. Some may want to find other people who understand how having the condition affects their lives. In contrast, others search for medical information, treatment options, the latest research, or financial aid resources. This information will help you learn more about the different information and services offered by nonprofit support and advocacy groups.

Nonprofit support and advocacy groups may be referred to as nonprofits, patient support groups, condition-specific organizations, advocacy groups, public charities, or registered charities. These terms tend to be used interchangeably rather than being specific to the group's focus. It is best to look beyond the label to find out what the group offers. I will refer to these groups as *nonprofit advocacy groups*.

These groups are primarily differentiated on the basis of their focus:

- *Condition-specific groups*: Many nonprofit advocacy groups focus on one rare or genetic condition or a group of closely related conditions, such as the Ehlers-Danlos Society or Dysautonomia International. Condition-specific groups often vary in their mission or focus. For example, some groups may focus on providing support or driving research, while other groups will offer a range of services, such as helping you find a doctor, organizing conferences, or working to gain the support of the local, state, or federal legislators.

- *Umbrella groups or alliances:* Nonprofit advocacy groups may join together to tackle more significant issues, such as advocating for legislation to help or protect all individuals with rare genetic conditions. One example of an umbrella group is the National Organization for Rare Disorders (NORD) at https://rarediseases.org/. These groups also may provide information and resources for specific medical conditions, but their activities and resources tend to focus more on helping the rare disease community.

- *General support groups:* Some groups focus on a symptom with many different causes, such as vision loss or developmental disabilities. Other groups may focus on the part of the body or a body system, such as the liver or the immune system. These groups tend to offer general information and resources that may help anyone dealing with challenges addressed by the group. For example, the Center for Parent Information and Resources (www.parentcenterhub.org) provides services to any family who has a child with disabilities.

Nonprofit advocacy groups typically offer the following types of services (individual groups may not provide all of these services, so it is essential to check each group's website or contact them to learn more about what they offer).

- *Support:* These groups help people connect with each other. Ways to connect online may include Facebook, blogs, listservs, Yahoo groups, and Twitter chats. Groups may provide opportunities to meet in person at yearly conferences, summer camps, or local meetings. Whether in person or online, support from others can empower you to take charge of your health.

- *Medical information:* Most groups provide medical information in easy-to-understand terms to help you learn more about your medical condition, available treatment options, and current research. Information is often on the group's website and may be available by mail, phone, or email. If you do call and leave a voicemail or send an email, keep in mind that many groups have minimal staff, so it may take a few days to get a reply.

- *Resources:* Nonprofit advocacy groups often have a list of helpful resources, such as related nonprofit advocacy groups, financial assistance resources, and sources for special medical equipment. They may be able to advise dealing with school or health insurance issues.

- *List of doctors or clinics:* Groups can have a list of medical care professionals and clinics to help you find specialists with experience in diagnosing or treating a rare medical condition. Groups may work closely with clinical centers, sometimes called Centers of Excellence, or be involved in the training of specialists. Many groups also have a medical advisory board made up of experts. If you can't find this information on the group's website, call or email the group to see if they can provide you with a list of doctors or clinics.

- *Registry:* A registry collects data about individuals, usually focused on a specific diagnosis or medical condition. Nonprofit advocacy groups maintain many rare disease registries to help advance medical research for a particular medical condition. If the group does not have its own disease registry, it may know an appropriate registry for your medical condition.

- *Research and clinical trials:* Clinical trials are medical research studies where people participate as volunteers. These studies may be evaluating new treatments or medications, searching for the cause(s) of a medical condition, or researching how the symptoms of the condition change over a person's lifetime. Whether you are interested in enrolling in a clinical trial or aim to stay aware of potential new treatments and advances, you may want to find a nonprofit advocacy group that provides information about the latest medical research. Some groups raise money to offer grants to medical researchers or pharmaceutical companies developing new treatments. Often these groups will keep data on their website about the progress of supported research.

- *Advocacy:* Advocacy for a rare medical condition may involve educating the public or medical community about the disease. A group may also take issues to local, state, and federal governments to pass legislation that will improve the lives of those affected by rare and genetic conditions.

Evaluating a group is not always easy. When you are looking for a nonprofit advocacy group, you want to make sure that the group offers helpful and up-to-date information. The group's mission statement can help you understand the focus of the group's activities. Also, look at who is involved in running the group. The group's staff members may have the medical condition themselves or have an affected family member. Other staff members may have a degree in a related field, such as social work, public health, education, communication, or medicine.

One word of caution when you seek out support groups—sometimes the occasional individual is not always supportive. I realize this sounds counterintuitive, but sometimes groups contain people who are suffering and talk about their struggles to the extent that it sometimes causes a downward spiral into a web of sadness for other members. It's okay to vent, and we all need validations from time to time, but try to seek out uplifting individuals that inspire and educate you and do not just commiserate.

The following list of nonprofit organizations is exceptional in helping you find hEDS support, research, education, and even good doctor lists. *Note:* The following list is always changing and difficult to maintain.

Ehlers-Danlos Society
1732 1st Ave. #20373
New York, NY 10128
Telephone: 410-670-7577
Email:info@ehlers-danlos.com ,
https://www.ehlers-danlos.com/eds-helpline/
Website: https://www.ehlers-danlos.com/

Ehlers-Danlos Support UK
PO Box 748
Borehamwood, WD6 9HU United Kingdom
Toll-free: 0800 907 8518 (in the UK)
Telephone: 0208 736 5604

Email: director@ehlers-danlos.org
Website: https://www.ehlers-danlos.org/

Hypermobility Syndromes Association (HMSA)
49 Greek Street
London, WD1 4EG United Kingdom,
Telephone: 033 3011 6388
Email: http://hypermobility.org/contact-us/
Website: http://hypermobility.org/

The Zebra Network
1122 Kenilworth Drive
Suite 307
Towson, MD 21204
Telephone: 410-825-0995
Email: victoria@thezebranetwork.org
Website: http://thezebranetwork.org/

Other EDS-related resources well worth your time to investigate include:

- **EDS Awareness** (http://www.chronicpainpart-ners.com/): Here you will find a geographic locator for support groups as well as medical practitioner webinars;

- **EDS Wellness** (http://www.edswellness.org/): Tons of video resources and interviews with specialists and other valuable resources available including EDS bootcamps;

- **Inspire** (https://www.inspire.com/): An online EDS support group forum sponsored by the EDS Society;

- **The ILC Foundation (Canada)** (http://www.theilcfoundation.org/category/eds): The "ILC" abbreviation is "Improving the Lives of Children" with the meaning of children of all ages including throughout adult life as hypermobile Ehlers-Danlos syndrome are affected at various times in life;

- **The Marfan Foundation** (http://www.marfan.org): A nonprofit organization that saves and improves lives while creating a community for all individuals with genetic aortic and vascular conditions, including Marfan, Loeys-Dietz, and Vascular Ehlers-Danlos syndromes;

- **Dysautonomia International** (http://dysautonomiainternational.org): A nonprofit that seeks to improve the lives of individuals living with autonomic nervous system disorders through research, physician education, public awareness, and patient empowerment programs;

- **Bobby Jones Chiari & Syringomyelia Foundation** (http://bobbyjonescsf.org): A nonprofit committed to advancing knowledge through research and to educate the medical, allied sciences, and lay

community about Chiari malformation, syringomyelia, and related disorders;

- **The Mast Cell Disease Society** (http://www.tms-forcure.org): A nonprofit organization dedicated to providing multifaceted support to patients, families, and medical professionals in our community and to leading the advancement of knowledge and research in mast cell diseases through education, advocacy, and collaboration;

- **Patient Advocacy Foundation** (https://www.patientadvocate.org/explore-our-resources/national-financial-resource-directory/): Promotes access to affordable, quality health care for people with chronic, debilitating, or life-threatening illnesses.

Social media

Social media sites can be a great (and free) way to connect peer-to-peer for support from anywhere (including a doctor's office waiting room), especially if a medical condition is very rare. You can try searching the condition name on platforms such as Facebook, Twitter, YouTube, Clubhouse, Discord, Telegram, Signal, Instagram, RareConnect, or WeChat to find a group (some require membership). The EDS Society offers a messaging forum to participate in at Inspire.com. If you want to set up your own community, Facebook offers training on how to utilize their platform to build your own that includes options for learning about messaging, polls, sharing of stories, and creating a place to ask questions of like-minded members that you moderate and/or administrate. You can share content for special events or days such as Rare Disease Day, or in May for EDS Awareness Month.

For any social media use, plan ahead and consider your goals, time you can invest, and understand each platform's features and risks. Be aware of your privacy preferences when sharing private health information online. If sharing sensitive info, use the pre-text "TRIGGER WARNING" for other users. Avoid ableist language or "inspiration porn" and always be inclusive. Trolling can happen when others have extreme responses to other people's posts. Handle them effectively in your own groups so as not to amplify their voice and keep the space safe.

Social media can be a great place to find fellow zebras, but medical information and advice that is offered by others is usually not reviewed by medical professionals, so caution is in order. Be conscious of your responsibilities for managing a group and liabilities in posting medical information.

Interviews with advocacy leaders

I interviewed several nonprofit advocacy group leaders to contribute their insights to the book, including major organizations helping with EDS, POTS, and CCI. Their collective wisdom can help you not just better understand the disorders, complexities, and research happening so you can make knowledgeable decisions about your care but also support you during this stressful time. You can find those interviews in the Appendix.

I had the privilege of doing a Q&A with the president of Dysautonomia International, Lauren Stiles. She

LAUREN STILES, CO-FOUNDER AND PRESIDENT OF DYSAUTONOMIA INTERNATIONAL

"I wish that all hypermobile EDS patients knew that POTS is not a life sentence. There is no doubt it is very difficult living with EDS and any form of dysautonomia, but there are people with hypermobile EDS and POTS who get better over time, and some fully recover from their POTS. A big myth in the patient community is that if you have hypermobile EDS and POTS, you'll never get better. We know that's not true, because we know patients with EDS and POTS who got dramatically better, and some who considered themselves recovered from POTS, even though they still have EDS."

was remarkably engaging and hopeful about the promise of upcoming research. Read the plans for the future of the organization in the full transcript of our conversation on my website at www.holdingitalltogether.com.

I also had the opportunity to interview the president of the Ehlers-Danlos Society, Lara Bloom, to talk about

LARA BLOOM, PRESIDENT OF THE EHLERS DANLOS SOCIETY

"It's misleading to a lot of EDSers who get a diagnosis and then become very worried that they're going to get all of the different comorbidities. That's simply not true. There's a big spectrum of EDS and HSD, and people are affected in different ways. It's also important to remember you don't have to have all the comorbidities and all the issues to get a diagnosis."

her plans for the future of the organization. My website at www.holdingitalltogether.com also has a full transcript of our conversation.

Finally, I had the opportunity to interview the executive director of the nonprofit Bobby Jones Chiari & Syringomyelia Foundation (CSF), Dorothy Poppe, to talk

DOROTHY POPPE, EXECUTIVE DIRECTOR OF THE BOBBY JONES CHIARI & SYRINGOMYELIA FOUNDATION

"We have to listen to the patients, but we also have to listen to the neurosurgeons because they're grappling with a lot of these things, too. When we go into a meeting, it's hearing what issues and obstacles doctors also face in treatment technology and more to bring this together. And we hear what difficulties they're going to have if they do research studies or what they need and what do the patients need? I think of our organization as the glue that brings those two things together, and that makes for success."

about the focus of the organization. The full transcript of our conversation can be found on my website at www. holdingitalltogether.com.

Medical research information

These resources provide more information about disease. The in-depth resources contain medical and scientific language that may be hard to understand. You may want to review these resources with a medical professional.

- **MedlinePlus** (http://www.nlm.nih.gov/medlineplus/ency/article/001468.htm): Designed by the National Library of Medicine to help you research your health questions.

- **Genetics Home Reference (GHR)** (http://ghr.nlm.nih.gov/condition=ehlersdanlossyndrome): Contains information on hEDS. This website is maintained by the National Library of Medicine.

- **The National Organization for Rare Disorders (NORD)** (http://www.rarediseases.org/rare-disease-information/rare-diseases/byID/240/viewAbstract): Has a report for patients and families about hEDS.

- **Mendeley** (https:www.mendeley.com): An online research search tool for academic papers.

In-depth medical information can be found at the following sites:

- **GeneReviews** (http://www.ncbi.nlm.nih.gov/bookshelf/br.fcgi?book=gene&part=eds3): This group provides current, expert-authored, peer-reviewed, full-text articles describing the application of genetic testing to the diagnosis, management, and genetic counseling of patients with specific inherited conditions.

- **Medscape Reference** (http://reference.medscape.com/multispecialty): This site provides information on this topic (you may need to register to view the medical textbook, but registration is free).

  - **Clinical Presentation of Ehlers-Danlos Syndrome** http://emedicine.medscape.com/article/1114004-overview): Here is an EDS overview from Medscape Reference.

- **MeSH®** (Medical Subject Headings) (https://meshb.nlm.nih.gov/record/ui?ui=D004535): This is a terminology tool used by the National Library of Medicine.

- **Monarch Initiative** (https://monarchinitiative.org/disease/OMIM:130020): They bring together data about conditions from humans and other species to help physicians and biomedical researchers. Monarch's tools are designed to make it easier to compare the signs and symptoms (phenotypes) of different diseases and discover common features. This initiative is a collaboration between several academic institutions across the world and is funded by the National Institutes of Health.

- **Online Mendelian Inheritance in Man (OMIM)** (http://www.omim.org/130020): This site is a catalog of human genes and genetic disorders. Each entry has a summary of related medical articles. It is meant for health care professionals and researchers.

- **Orphanet** (http://www.orpha.net): Access to this European database reference portal for information on rare diseases and orphan drugs is free of charge.

- **PubMed** (https://pubmed.ncbi.nlm.nih.gov/): A searchable database of medical literature and lists journal articles that discuss Hypermobile Ehlers-Danlos syndrome.

- **NORD's Organizational Database (ODB)** (https://rarediseases.org/for-patients-and-families/connect-others/find-patient-organization/): This database was established to provide organizations and resources for patients and families affected by rare diseases. Organizations can be included in the ODB if they provide free information and/or services helpful to individuals and families affected by one or more rare diseases, have a website, are non-commercial, are transparent regarding sponsors or sources of funding, and are transparent regarding sources and/or reviewers of medical information provided on their websites and/or publications.

- **GenomeConnect** (https://www.clinicalgenome.org/genomeconnect/for-patients-genomeconnect/): This site is an online tool people can use to share their genetic test results and health information with researchers and health care providers. You can also connect with other individuals who have a similar diagnosis or related symptoms.

- **MyGene2** (https://www.mygene2.org/MyGene2/): Similar to GenomeConnect, MyGene2 is an online tool that families interested in sharing their health and genetic information can use to connect with other families, clinicians, and researchers.

- **RareConnect** (https://www.rareconnect.org/en/communities): This site has online communities for patients and families with rare medical conditions so they can connect with others and share their experiences.

- **RareShare** (https://rareshare.org/): This site too offers an online social hub dedicated to patients, families, and health care professionals who are affected by rare medical disorders.

- **DNAandU.org** (https://www.dnaandu.org/): A website and blog that collects firsthand stories from people making tough decisions about using genomic (DNA) information in their own health care choices.

Choose to Assess, Act, or Affirm

- **Assess:** Determine three new resources can you utilize to further your understanding of EDS from the list.

- **Act:** Search for social media groups, community forums in Discord, or in apps such as *The Zebra Club* to connect with others.

- **Affirm:** "My diagnosis was the starting point to build a better life. I am willing to believe in my ability to create healing and happiness."

Bibliography

"Support for Patients and Families | Genetic and Rare." https://rarediseases.info.nih.gov/guides/pages/120/support-for-patients-and-families.

"Support for patients and families—GARD-PRP Survival Guide." https://prpsurvivalguide.org/support-for-patients-and-families-gard/.

NOTES

MAKING IT

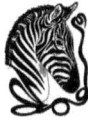

Examine and define your values. Really. What do you want for your life? How do you want to feel? What sort of life will allow you to feel at peace at the end of your lifetime? How would you live if you lived with no regrets? This is not a task-oriented "Bucket List." This is a way to have the sort of life you want to identify what grounds you and guides you.

—Angela Marchesani

Several elements are vital to making it with EDS or any chronic illness. In my opinion, it comes down to making moments and making it happen while remembering that you are not alone in your struggle.

Making moments

I have a sign in my bedroom I see every day that says, "Collect memories, not things." Making moments and memories is one of the most important activities I focus my time on. These will last a lifetime. Making memories can be something silly like dancing in the rain together, going to scary movies and jumping out of the seat together, or cooking a great meal together at home and having fun when you didn't burn it this time. You need to take time to make memories with the people you love and care for, whether your friends, family, and those you choose as your family. Life is the culmination of all of our experiences—invest wisely.

I also try to take trips and vacations to experience new things and cultures and meet new people. This is essential to reclaim the world as yours after being diagnosed with a chronic illness such as EDS. While out in the world experiencing the newness, I would often get some form of a small physical memento or souvenir to cherish and remind me of those times. It's important that it was a memento of the experience instead of a thing to own. I have a collection of simple pieces of jewelry that I've collected around the world and look at them daily to reexperience the gifts I received during those joyous times.

You also can hold on to good times to keep yourself positively focused by creating scrapbooks or photo memory albums. I like to use the simplicity of today's Internet tools to upload pictures and easily design and create coffee table books that I browse regularly. I am invited back into the memory by viewing the images, and it's like a mini vacation all over again for my brain. As memory and cognition can fade with age and chronic illness, scrapbooks give you a great way to recall happy moments. Having struggled with cognitive decline and memory loss, I am grateful to have memory books of my photos to bring back all the good times on a rough day.

Making it happen

They say 80 percent of life is showing up. Success with a chronic illness then is being there and showing up for yourself. if you don't show up for yourself, you can't be there for anyone else. That is the lesson to learn. You have to come first. You are the person for whom you need to make things happen. That means not just making a plan but taking action steps toward making that plan happen. That builds momentum in ways that will lead to success.

Everyone will make things happen for themselves differently. Maybe you are an avid researcher and have helped people in your journey to improve their life by sharing information on your disease. Maybe you have become a patient advocate. And maybe it's just enough right now for you to get out of bed this morning. No matter what you do, you are engrossed in a lifelong project of dealing with EDS.

If everyone with EDS came together to share resources, knowledge, symptom-tracking tools, and much more, the world of hypermobility and its unknowns would explode with positive energy and leapfrog forward in terms of treatment. You can join local and online forums or groups of like-minded fellow zebras to get support, you can educate your loved ones on what hEDS is, and you can fight your own bold fight in your own way. No matter what you choose, find a purpose in having this disease by sharing what you know. Or as Nelson Mandela said, "May your choices reflect your hopes, not your fears."

You are not alone

I don't know why, but knowing that I'm not alone in facing EDS makes me feel just a little bit better. It turns out that there are even celebrities with EDS. I had the pleasure to interview fellow zebra Camille Schrier, Miss America 2020. In 2019, Camille was selected Miss Virginia after breaking tradition to perform a really engaging educational science demonstration. She went on to win Miss America later that year as the only woman to have ever had science help her with her talent performance as she did an experiment rather than dancing, singing, or performing. I wanted to know how she copes, what she has done to raise awareness, and how we might support each other as a community. (The full transcript can be found with the audio on my website at www.holdingitalltogether.com.)

When were you diagnosed with EDS?

- "I always had signs that pointed to joint hypermobility, and Ehlers-Danlos Syndrome from the day I was born. And it took 11 years for us to figure out that that was what I was dealing with. It's pretty interesting because I want to say there's a statistic that says it takes between 12 to 13 years for a patient who first exhibits symptoms to actually be diagnosed with EDS. This was kind of true for me because I was born with my hips dislocated. That was the first symptom of EDS. And throughout my childhood, I always got hurt. I always bruised. I was always kind of clumsy."

What has had the biggest impact in your life having EDS?

- "The biggest part of this entire story for me is the early diagnosis compared to my mom's later diagnosis. I think that watching my mom struggle with chronic pain, surgeries, injuries, steroid injections and going through her own spinal fusion and rotator cuff injuries. She had so many things going on when she didn't know that she had this problem. That could have potentially prevented a lot of the injuries in her life that I have the opportunity to do as a young person who knows that I have the diagnosis."

How did you compete while you suffered from EDS?

- "When I decided to compete for Miss America and Miss Virginia, I was most concerned about how I would be able to maintain the role with the fatigue that I experience. I wasn't so much worried about the pain and everything else that I'm now experiencing now, but just being able to do the job. I experience brain fog and this exhaustion level that wouldn't necessarily be rectified with sleep. And frankly, being Miss America is not a restful job. The job is really traveling 20,000 miles a month, moving hotels every night, every day to a new location, and being 'on' the whole day."

You were the first Miss America to serve during a pandemic. What was that like?

- "I was able to travel virtually throughout the country by sitting at my desk and logging in to Zoom. I was able to create videos that live on forever. I did a whole series with PBS here in central Virginia, and it was called 'Cooking Up Science with Miss America.' Projects like that allowed me to do the job that I wanted to do and make the impact that I wanted to make without taxing my body in the way that a traditional Miss America would have had to do. And for that, I'm really grateful. And a lot of people who are very big fans of Miss America will assume or ask me about am I disappointed in my experience? I'm absolutely not. I couldn't be any more grateful for the way that my job changed as a person with a chronic illness, to allow me to serve that role in a way that worked for my body in such a serendipitous way. To be able to focus on science because that was the way that I got my job and then to be able to advocate for science and science education during a pandemic was just the perfect fit. That's how I've done Miss America with EDS."

What was the best thing you got to do as Miss America?

- "The most fun thing that I got to do was go on a USO tour. Like the Bob Hope USO tours that happened for so long, those still continue. I went with the vice chairman of the Joint Chiefs of Staff, and we did a ten-day excursion throughout the United States and went to Cuba as well visiting military service members and their families. Because we were on domestic soil, there were a lot of families and kids there. We were able to really understand more about what military service looks like and I think for a lot of the members that was just such an incredible trip to go on. It is an iconic Miss America trip that has existed since Vietnam. I got to be a little part of history."

The list of people with hEDS is staggering, but maybe it will lead to better awareness and resources to come. Actresses Lena Dunham and Jameela Jamil and pop singer song artist Sia and Halsey have also publicly said they suffer from hEDS. There are many theories that Elvis struggled with hypermobile EDS and chronic pain. I also read that Elizabeth Taylor and President Abe Lincoln had it too (but I have no evidence). Medical professionals now say that 1 in 500 people can have hEDS. Maybe it's no longer rare but just rarely diagnosed!

But getting that diagnosis is vital. Data now say it averages 14 years for an EDS patient to be correctly diagnosed. But that's when the magic happens when you get a proper diagnosis, then there are the joys of having a name for what you have! You can start researching and finally get some validation for your sense of loss and emptiness and find others who also struggle who can be compassionate. Even more importantly, you may find a care team member who can start treating you to improve your well-being.

Final thoughts

Life isn't exactly a predictable affair. Sooner or later, everyone faces adversity. Developing your habit of expanding your comfort zone equips you to better handle change and ambiguity with more poise, leading to enhanced resilience.

Living with chronic illness can be stressful, but you can take steps to manage your condition and maintain a good quality of life. Learn as much as you can about your illness and treatment needs. Be proactive about following your treatment plan, and lead a healthy lifestyle. Face your pain and your fears about it, and come to acceptance. Make time for activities and relationships that leave you feeling happier and supported while avoiding people and things that stress you out. Manage the complications, emergencies, and risk as best you can. Make future choices that will suit your new lifestyle and habits.

To that end, I suggest you take any of the tips that resonate with you in this book and write them down now in a journal or on a piece of paper that you can have in front of you to post on the refrigerator. Practice any of the healing habits to help you become the person you want to be.

The road to resilience is long, but you can reclaim your life on your own if you are tenacious about it. If you can figure out *why* you want your life back, let that motivate you to learn *how*. You can improve your ability to live a better life. May we all be capable of change. You can change your ability to live a better life. Let's all try to be a little better than we used to be.

Remember, you are rare. You are a zebra. You are like a diamond, formed in the harsh circumstances of becoming who and what you are, and you can shine brilliantly. This journey is up to you! You have the choice to make a change in your own life. I know it sounds like rainbows and unicorns, but you have more control over your brain's neuroplasticity than you realize. Life is not always perfect, but you can make progress, and you are worth it.

A final word of advice: take it easy on yourself. Rest up, be well, and remember to be mindful that you are an incredible healing being. It is easier to embrace the journey itself and take your happiness from there. You now know the steps and have been given a handful of tips to get you started on the right foot. Now is the time to change for the better!

IF YOU CAN ONLY RECALL A FEW THINGS FROM THIS BOOK, TRY TO HOLD ONTO THESE THINGS:

Perseverance is the key. Stay on the journey to joy, never give up, roll with the tide, and prepare yourself to see all of the diamond's beautiful facets that are forming within you. All aspects will shine and show its beauty in its rarity. Write down your dreams, your rights, your wish list, why you want to change, and then how you are going to do it. Action creates a reaction.

Your pain is not your identity. Being a chronically ill person is not your identity. You are a great human being first, who happens to have health issues. You can break the pain-fear cycle.

Chaos within can change into self-compassion. As you know, change is the only constant in life, so learn to go with the flow, adapt, and change. Get unstuck. My parents have been giving me this advice for decades, but I finally learned the lesson when facing this health crisis.

You do you and learn to let the rest go. Remember, we all are created equal. The process of coming to terms with accepting living with chronic illness is long, challenging, and takes a great deal of time and patience. You will have hills and valleys along the path. You will need to grieve. With acceptance then comes healing. Many people say that following the 12 steps of Alcoholic Anonymous can be helpful to rebuild your life from scratch. Believe there is infinite hope. Nurture it.

Choose joy every day and live your life to the fullest as nothing but your true authentic self. Get enthusiastic about rebuilding, reprogramming, and restoring as you are the only one who is responsible and accountable for your own self and your thinking. This is programming. You can rewire your negativity bias. Where your energy goes, growth flows.

Give yourself peace and grace. Namaste. Have the goal of peace and calm in your life and work hard to protect it. Live with no regrets. Live for what you have, not what you want. Live like every day could be your last because as you face your chronic illness like I face mine, we know every day counts. Cherish it.

For what it's worth…
It's never too late, or in my case, too early.
To be whoever we want to be.
There's no time limit.
Start whenever you want.
You can change or stay the same.
There are no rules to this thing.
We can make the best of it.
I hope you see things
That startle you.
I hope you feel things
You never felt before.
I hope you meet people who
Have a different point of view.
I hope you live a life
You're proud of,
And if you're not,
I hope you have the courage
To start all over again.

—Olivia Rose

ABOUT THE AUTHOR

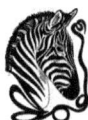

I lost my most important asset—my health. They say, "When you don't have your health, you've got nothing." Right? It is true, and all zebras know it. We can feel lost. But you are not alone.

I spent several years learning to be able to climb. First to be able to climb the stairs in my home again, then climb out of my walker. I started to rise up, slowly, stronger. Researching voraciously how to heal anyway I could. With a patience I had never possessed before, I found the resilience and courage to choose to become the hero of my own life and learned how to practice wellness and discover I could choose joy where I found purpose and fulfillment.

I am now certified to teach, mentor, and advocate for others on the topics of life purpose, life optimization, positive psychology, mindfulness, qigong, and tai chi mindful movement. I was also trained by the Ehlers-Danlos Society's ECHO program in EDS patient advocacy.

I have been formally trained to run chronic pain-related support groups for the US Pain Foundation. As I finish this manuscript, I am training to hopefully get back to work as a patient advocate to help others more formally get the best from our medical system in terms of costs and care.

I am not a licensed therapist or health care provider but a mentor, guide, and advocate—a fellow chronic illness sufferer who serves as an accountability partner. I have turned my personal tragedy into triumph and gone from exhausted to exuberant. I hope you fellow chronically ill sufferers can also choose to make a change, have the courage to see it through to action, and live with purpose and the ends in mind. Life is short. Make it what you want *now*. Live in the present and appreciate all of the abundance we still have. Life is about being present, not perfect.

Can I help you navigate the journey?

Our personal growth can feel a lot like climbing a steep mountain. It is a struggle, and it is hard to know the next steps. I approach my clients with a view of a Sherpa or guide. Mountain climbers face massive challenges on their journey. Because the mountain is steep and rugged, it is hard to see where they are going. It is also hard to get good handholds and footholds in the rock face.

I see the process of helping others as a fellow mountain climber. From my vantage point, I can see where you came from, where you are going, and what your next handhold and foothold could be. I can give you feedback about what

I see next for you on your journey. I might see more clearly where you are getting stuck and give you some ideas about your next steps.

To learn more, connect with me or check out my free courses available at my business website www.journey-2joyous.com or access resources mentioned within this book at www.holdingitalltogether.com. Follow me on social media or subscribe to my newsletters for information, insights, and inspiration on living well with chronic illness, including hypermobile Ehlers-Danlos syndrome. I offer patient advocacy, support, guidance, and more. Feel free to contact me directly at cchypermobile@gmail.com.

Follow me on social

- **Facebook:** Christie Calm – https://www.facebook.com/christie.calm.5/
- **Instagram:** Christie Cox Calm – https://www.instagram.com/christiecoxcalm/
- **YouTube:** Journey2Joy – https://www.youtube.com/channel/UChiqso6PhnX39eODTVHqRhw
- **Twitter:** https://twitter.com/joy_journey2
- **Inspire:** https://www.inspire.com/m/christie_calm/
- **Pinterest:** @journey2joyous – https://pin.it/6sEL1Tn
- **TikTok:** https://www.tiktok.com/@ccalm123

HEALTH CARE HEROES

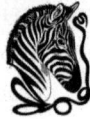

Many of you may be familiar with the American TV show *House*, starring a uniquely inquisitive doctor as the strange, drug-addicted, quirky yet brilliant healer. The main character is Dr. Gregory House (played by Hugh Laurie) as an unconventional, misanthropic medical genius who, despite his dependence on pain medication, leads a team of diagnosticians in a fictional hospital with regular rare disease patients who are always amazingly diagnosed within the 60-minute program.

Finding your way through the health care system isn't like that—at all. Living with EDS can be daunting. Many health insurance companies confine your choices to a narrow panel of doctors or therapists. I do not believe the medical care system, particularly in the United States, is set up correctly to provide the care in health care. It is set up to make money for insurance companies and elitists. There is nothing about health or care. It is about sickness and turning a profit. Many people say it is a broken system. But it is working exactly as the people designed it to work and not always for the benefit of patients.

However, there are exceptions, and a few inspirational care providers are available and working hard to help patients. I am fortunate enough to have researched voraciously to find the best care team possible, and I want to share their wisdom with you in the pages that follow.

I am honored to have had the opportunity to interview and share the wisdom of a few of my care team members below, who I call my Health Care Heroes. There are tips from an ophthalmologist from Johns Hopkins, a hypermobile expert in physical therapy, an EDS-knowledgeable neurosurgeon, and others. I hope these interviews firmly implant the theme that is key to my lessons in this book—that it takes a village to care for EDS. By that I mean it takes you going to several multidisciplinary types of doctors and specialists to form a holistic view of how you are doing, your symptoms, and to manage your ongoing care.

With the exceptional care of my Health Care Heroes, I have moved from a level of disability now to a greater quality of life and being more enabled. I am very grateful for their care and their gracious time to pass on wisdom.

My neuro-ophtalmologist: Dr. Eric Singman

Many people with EDS struggle with their vision, seeing double, convergence and balance issues that a neuro-ophtalmologist can assist with.

Dr. Singman specializes in neuro-ophthalmology with a particular interest in the effects of brain injury on vision. As such, he has seen many patients with Ehlers-Danlos because they appear to be more susceptible to trauma and less able to recover as quickly or completely as normal. I interviewed him in August 2021 for this book. See my website for the full transcript. Below are a few highlights.

How do you approach patients you suspect might be hypermobile when doing their neurological vision exam?

- **Dr. Singman:** "I do a full spectrum review of multi-system symptoms including looking for the following common symptoms I have seen in my practice":
  - Mast cells;
  - Dysautonomia;
  - Gastrointestinal issues;
  - Craniocervical instability and/or Chiari;
  - Hernia;
  - Fatigue and sleep issues;
  - Prolapse;
  - Teeth grinding (bruxism);
  - Neck problems;
  - Brain fog.

> "Sometimes I feel like the best question to ask is, '*Where doesn't it hurt?*'" says Dr. Singman

"I use the Beighton score to give me an idea of hyper-mobility and then offer a full eye exam. No EDS patient wants to hear, 'How do you feel so bad when you look so good?' as that dismissal so commonly seen in the medical community can crush a patient. If the patient has confirmed hEDS, then depending upon what resources they have built around themselves, I often refer them to other specialists which can be very hard to get in to see. If they have potential Chiari or craniocervical instability, I immediately order an MRI, upright not supine, with flexion and extension. It seems to be a more effective way to detect that."

What common comorbidities and conditions do you also find in EDSrs?

- **Dr. Singman:** "One of the things I look for as an ophthalmologist is the diagnosis of convergence insufficiency, a condition where you have reduced endurance for near vision work. I give these patients online exercises through two different programs, one called HTS, one called Vizual Edge. These programs slowly build visual motor skills, take very little investment, and you can do it anytime, anywhere."

You have a great deal of understanding and compassion for EDSrs. Why is that?

- **Dr. Singman:** "EDSs patients are frankly more fragile, easily breakable, and need more care. The story of a Ming vase is like an EDS patient—they're fragile—but they're often perfect until they experience trauma. The medical community needs to treat them as such."

My Physical therapist: Dr. Amanda Miller, PT, DPT, WCS

Many people with EDS need physical therapy to build strength and keep injuries and joints stabilized.

Below are the key highlights from my interview with my physical therapist who has a specialty in hypermobile patients, specifically women with pelvic floor issues, Dr. Amanda Miller from Progress Physical Therapy.

What is your area of specialty within PT?

- **Amanda Miller:** "One group I see a lot of has been diagnosed as IBS (irritable bowel syndrome), so either constipation, diarrhea or mixed or just abdominal pain that leads to dysfunction, difficulty with eating and then dysfunctional motility. A large component of my practice is looking specifically at the pelvic floor. If a patient has underlying weakness in pelvic floor, transverse abdominis, and you combine that with somebody who has EDS or hypermobility, it sets you up for muscle overactivity or spasm, especially for my EDS pregnant or postpartum clients. What that looks like with those patients is usually pelvic girdle or pelvic floor muscle pain. So that could be pelvic pain, pubic pain, SI joint pain, pain with intercourse, difficulty emptying their bowel, difficulty emptying their bladder or urinary, urgency, frequency, that kind of thing. And that's how pelvic health really ties in with EDS, especially because pelvic health encompasses prenatal and postpartum. Those EDS folks are especially at risk of injury and pain."

What have you learned from your EDS patients?

- **Amanda Miller:** "It's very important to make sure that you're not changing too much too quickly, and that what you are doing is in line with what the patient wants to do. I've got some EDS patients who are preparing for pregnancy, and that's one area of focus, and then I've got others who are marathon runners, and so we have to focus on different things and then others still who are just trying to be able to sit at their office job comfortably. So it's important that I make sure that I am considering the patient's needs and the individuality of the patient when I'm making our plans of care and doing our treatment. And then, of course, being super flexible because there's usually a lot of symptoms with EDS patients. It's a lot of ups and downs and we have to adjust our treatment plan, almost every visit."

What advice do you have for women considering childbirth to ensuring their pelvic health?

- **Amanda Miller:** "If you plan to have children as a person with EDS, you should be going to PT first. You should think about doing a "pre-hab" program, to prepare you for pregnancy and then work with a PT during pregnancy and then, of course continue during the postpartum period. If you're going through menopause, that's something to prepare for that can change your muscle health and strength. I think when you have chronic musculoskeletal dysfunction, you should plan on having annual PT visits anyway."

Any other comments or anything you want to share with the EDS community?

- **Amanda Miller:** "I think the most important thing is just to be proactive. Be as proactive as possible. When I look at my patients who have had a lot of success with their care versus the ones who have not, it's the ones that are very proactive that do better. Preventative care and strength building is important."

My neurosurgeon: Dr. Sunil Patel, Chief of Neurosurgery at MUSC

Patients with joint instability in the spine should see a neurologist and if necessary, a neurosurgeon for evaluation.

I interviewed Dr. Patel following my recovery from my surgery, and we caught up in January 2022. Below are a few of the highlights; read the full very informative interview transcript on my website.

Can you tell me about your experience with EDS patients and the complexities that we typically face?

- **Dr. Patel:** "EDS is a complex disorder, not as well understood as it should be, however becoming more recognized by a variety of specialists. Ehlers and Danlos originally described this syndrome of collagen, or connective tissue disorder many decades ago, and the criteria for who has EDS or who doesn't have also evolved quite a bit. We now know that there are 13 different types of EDS and probably the most common form of EDS, which is still under recognized, is what we call hypermobile EDS or type three EDS. While we know that there are familial tendencies with it and therefore there's probably a genetic inheritance of this disorder, that genetic inheritance still remains to be defined. Our Norris Lab at MUSC is working on finding this genetic source. Every organ, tendon, muscle, bone, blood vessel and your skin has collagen. You can imagine that if you have something different about the collagen as in type three EDS (or hypermobile EDS) patients, that the systemic manifestations can be different in different patients and involve a lot of different symptoms. My engagement with treating EDS patients is because of their spinal manifestations. By that I mean the laxity of the

ligament affects the function of the spine and therefore affects the nervous system, the spinal cord and
nerves. Every spinal joint, from your head to your
sacrum, can be affected. The lax ligaments and
softened intervertebral discs cause hypermobility
at each of the segments—what some of us refer to
as instability. In your case, it was a cranio-cervical
instability. In this situation the ligaments holding
the skull to the top of the spinal bones are lax, or
like 'rubber bands' rather than being non-elastic.
This results in a hypermobility of that joint, and
that leads to symptoms of pain and strain on the
neck muscles. But more importantly, it affects the
spinal cord and or medulla within canal at the cervical junction and hence the neurological manifestations from that. When I see these patients, it's
very clear that their spine symptoms are not the
only ones that they suffer from. They have different
organ system problems – cardiovascular symptoms
like POTS or GI symptoms from hypermobility or
hyperfunction of the gut or the stomach, gastric
emptying problems. There seems to be an unexplained prevalence of Mast cell activation syndrome
in hEDS patients—a dysfunction of Mast cells
which is one of the immune cells in our body. How
all these things are linked with each other is not
yet known. I'm sure once we figure out the genetic
code or the gene defects, we will be able to better

understand the pathophysiology of all these organ systems."

How would a person know to come see a neurosurgeon like you who understands EDS? What symptoms might they look for?

- **Dr. Patel:** "Symptoms can be neurological—like balance issues, brain fog, sensory motor symptoms in the arms and legs, cranial nerve symptoms, swallowing issues—and so on. Testing can help confirm the craniocervical instability (CCI) and I prefer two key imaging studies—an upright MRI of the cervical spine and x-rays with flexion and extension views. Sometimes I've used a cervical rotational CT scan to look for atlantoaxial instability (AAI). It's important to look at these dynamic imaging studies to objectively measure the abnormal motion between segments and the effect on the spinal cord. I think there's a reason why the average time to diagnosis of EDS is about 14 years per recent publications."

Do you believe that hypermobility is becoming more recognized?

- **Dr. Patel:** "I now see ten to 15 patients a week in my clinic sometimes, and it's quite overwhelming for me alone but I don't think the incidence has increased. I think the recognition of hypermobility has increased. In fact, there are now epidemiologic papers that show that maybe one in 500 people have it. I suspect this is conservative. That's startling! I think with all this statistical information, knowledge and better diagnostics and dissemination of knowledge, we're going to see more and more patients given this diagnosis and appropriately treated."

As I understand it, you, MUSC and your colleague Dr Norris are working to find the genetic marker which could bring a faster diagnosis for hypermobile EDS as a genetic disorder. What promises does that bring for patients?

- **Dr. Patel:** "Once you have a gene, you can do an early diagnosis where if a patient is not responding to standard treatments, for example, neck pain or spinal symptoms. They can get a simple genetic test—now that would be helpful. And in addition to that, knowing the presence of the genetic defect, in a parent who has hypermobility the provider can prepare the patients and perhaps test their children for earlier diagnosis and perhaps even intervention and even prevention of symptom manifestation."

How did you learn about EDS?

- **Dr Patel:** "Back in medical school 35 years ago, EDS was something I just memorized as a collagen disorder. And I got that question right on the exam, and that was the end of that. And it was thought to be a very rare collagen disorder, just like Marfans and a number of other collagen disorders. And I thought to myself then I said, well, this is rare. I'll never see it. But I got the question right. EDS, yes, Marfans, yes. And that was the end. Or so I thought. It was not very well known then and not recognized to be as common as it is today. I'm not an EDS expert. There's no such thing. You don't go to Med school and then you do a residency in EDS management. As I told you, EDS manifests itself in a lot of different organ systems. Nor is there a neurosurgery training, in which I did a special rotation during the seven years of training, saying, okay, this month you're going to see EDS patients. That doesn't exist. So how did I become the so-called expert? People call me the expert, but it's not that. I think it's my personal experience in practicing medicine that I always don't stick people on a shelf who come in with symptoms that I don't understand that sound real. When you start gathering more than five or ten of these patients with similar symptoms, nothing else seems to be working out. You pull those off the shelf and you say, there's something common about these people. They're not crazy and they're having real and common symptoms."

MUSC SCIENTISTS TACKLE EDS RESEARCH AND PROMISE HOPE

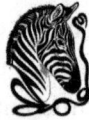

At the Medical University of South Carolina (MUSC), Dr. Russell "Chip" Norris, Cortney Gensemer PhD, and his team at their hEDS lab, called the Norris Lab, have created some very special momentum on EDS research as of the writing of this book.

I had the opportunity to watch a webinar hosted by the Washington, DC, Area EDS support group with EDS Wellness where they shared preliminary research findings including noting initial genetic markers in families and common demographic data. Watch the video here: https://www.youtube.com/watch?v=UF22V3Pw2p8. I also had the unique chance to interview them on Zoom for a Q&A in November 2021, which is highlighted below.

The Norris Lab hEDS patient registry started in 2020 and in one year they had about 900 participants who had shared their DNA samples to provide the data to lead MUSC's genetic research. Only a couple of years since inception, it now has thousands of patients and growing. If you want to help the future of research, consider joining the Norris Lab or fund their research with MUSC as they are doing great things to advance the diagnosis and treatment of hEDS. Watch for more from the Norris Lab on hypermobile EDS to come.

Dr. Chip Norris and Cortney Gensemer from MUSC

The following are a few highlights from our conversation, while the full transcript from the session where I interviewed their team leaders, Dr. Chip Norris and Cortney Gensemer, is available on my book website at www.holdingitalltogether.com.

Cortney, I understand that you have hypermobile EDS. Tell me about your experience.

- **Cortney:** "I was diagnosed with hEDS when I was in undergrad when I was around 19. I had never heard of it, but I had issues my whole life, and it is the kind of thing that connects all the dots and sort of makes everything make sense. I was a super competitive athlete, so I had a lot of injuries, and a lot of surgeries. But the EDS diagnosis has definitely changed the way I was living my life. I'm still dealing with some of those consequences before then, but I've been able to make better life decisions now that I know which is one of the reasons we advocate for earlier diagnosis."

MUSC and the Norris lab are doing exciting things. Tell me about what the lab is looking to research. What sorts of answers for EDS?

- **Cortney:** "I think that our accomplishments so far and all of the attention has been on finding a gene or genes for EDS, but that's really sort of the starting point. Genetics is where it's starting and the information we get from genetics, then we will look at biology to see what's actually happening as a consequence of that mutation to the connective tissues. And then hopefully, how can we use that information to make a diagnostic test. And how can we use that information to develop some sort of way to treat us. The big goal at the end of the day is finding a way to take this information and go back and help patients. But even a diagnostic test is huge, and I don't think adding it to a genetic panel, but even something simpler, like from a blood test or something that your primary care doctor or pediatrician can order and you get blood work done and, you know, definitively if you have this."

What do you hope genetic testing will help accomplish?

- **Dr. Norris:** "It's a challenge because there's a lot of information out there that's just not based in science. People who are just trying to learn more about it get inundated with stuff that they don't know what's right, they don't know what's wrong. And so really finding the right clinical care team is important that can give you the right scientifically and clinically sound advice."

- **Cortney:** "There are no clear guidelines out there. Okay, you have EDS and now this is what you do."

- **Dr. Norris:** "There are a lot of personal stories about things working, different things, working well for certain individuals that may not be relatable to across the board. And so one of the big challenges, as everybody knows, is consistency of care. And physicians don't know about this disease, or if they do, they read a paragraph when they were in Med school about it. There's not a standard. I think one of the things that we're trying to do through our clinical networks here is to establish some sort of standardized clinical management for hEDS so there'll be guidelines on what is actually scientifically valid to develop. It may not be a one size fits all, but it will be based in science in medicine."

What's the big audacious goal of your lab and the patient registry? What's going to be success for you?

- **Cortney:** "The Institute, combined with our research. We want EDS patients to be able to come here and see the geneticist, then they might need to see Dr Patel. They need to see orthopedics, they need to see different areas. They come here, they have those appointments, they get genetic testing while they're here. The testing is done by our lab. We get a skin biopsy or a biopsy from their shoulder surgery while they're here. And those contribute to our research. And that research is allowing us to diagnose patients and come up with treatment. Having that full circle system. That is the big goal."

- **Dr Norris:** "It would be amazing to go even a step further and have I mean, ideally, my big dream would be to develop an Institute, make it success-ful. Have people from all over the world come here. To be able to figure out how to make insurance plans work and then have a Ronald McDonald's type house, a subsidized housing situation available for patients to come to Charleston."

MAKING THE DECISION TO FILE FOR DISABILITY

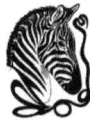

Deciding to file for disability through private insurance, such as an employer's Short Term Disability plan, or through the Social Security Administration (SSA), is a giant decision emotionally. It often means you have to accept that you are no longer capable of working and you have to give up your job or career, income, and ability to provide for yourself and your family. The ramifications of such a grand decision are countless and should be weighed accordingly. I strongly suggest you do your research before making a decision, and I recommend you consult with a disability attorney.

Social Security Administration Disability

If you have been diagnosed with an ongoing medical condition that affects your ability to work, then you've probably thought about applying for disability benefits. For someone unfamiliar with Social Security Disability Insurance (SSDI) and Supplemental Security Income (SSI), the application process can be daunting. You should apply for disability benefits as soon as possible once you're unable to work or maintain gainful employment as a result of your medical condition.

The first step is to talk to your doctor about your intention to file for disability. As part of the application, you will sign a release that allows the SSA to collect medication information from your practitioners. It is essential that you review your records to make sure they are correct and request your doctors make any corrections before sending information to SSA. You can submit your medical information to SSA while it is reviewing your application, and this may potentially reduce the time it takes SSA to process an application.

The SSA website is the first place to start on whether you qualify and how to apply for SSDI or SSI (https://www.ssa.gov/benefits/disability/qualify.html).   SSDI   is based on your earnings and how much you paid into the Social Security Trust Fund, while SSI is assistance for those with low incomes and few assets. A person can be eligible for both SSDI and SSI, and a key criterion is that a person must have a physical or psychological disability that prevents them from working earning what SSA considers Substantial Gainful Activity (SGA) for at least 12 months. For 2022, SGA is earning $1,350 per month, though if you are blind, SGA is $2,260.

INTENT TO FILE TOOL WITH SOCIAL SECURITY ADMINISTRATION

In April 2022 the Social Security Administration (SSA) launched a new tool (https://www.ssa.gov/benefits/ssi/start.html) people can use to tell SSA that they—or someone they are helping—wants to apply for Supplemental Security Income (SSI) and other benefits.

The process takes only 5–10 minutes and asks for basic information about the person who wants to apply for SSI. A Social Security representative will schedule an appointment and email the appointment information. In some cases, they may call you to schedule the appointment.

Using this tool documents intent to file an application and establishes a protective filing date. This date determines when payments can begin for approved applicants.

Certain third parties, such as parents of minor children, family members, representatives, or members of advocacy groups, can also use the tool to express interest about applying for SSI on behalf of someone they are helping. For those unable to use the tool, SSA will continue to establish the protective filing date based on a written statement of intent to apply or an oral inquiry about program eligibility.

This tool is part of SSA's commitment to expanding online services and making it easier for people who face service barriers to get the support they need.

Need help understanding the disability process? The Patient Advocate Foundation's comprehensive, on-demand *Disability Training Series* and consumer guidebook can help. Visit https://bit.ly/3iahNUx.

In any case, you may want to speak with a disability attorney or advocate for an assessment or for help applying, either through SSA or your private insurance. They can be an excellent resource when filing out applications, collecting and reviewing medical records, and keeping paperwork organized. You can start an application without an attorney or advocate, but you should consult one before you appeal any denial. For SSDI, attorneys are only paid if your application is approved, and then their fees are capped at $6,000 or 25 percent of back-pay, whichever is less.

Insights from a Disability Attorney

I had the privilege to interview one of the nation's top disability lawyers for the book, Ben Glass. Below are highlights from an interview with him as well as his insights on Long-Term Disability (LTD), tips for successful applications, and applying with diagnoses such as EDS and POTS.

Interview Highlights/Excerpts by Topic

For about 22 years, Ben Glass has focused more and more on disability claims, and today all of his personal work is in the world of long-term disability insurance claims.

Applying

"Most of our clients are people who have been productive in their lives. Something happens—either an accident, they get an actual injury or some sort of illness, everything from a cancer diagnosis to a brain tumor to fibromyalgia, chronic fatigue syndrome. Something happens to their lives, which now either limits or prevents them from doing the work they were born to do. Christie, most of our clients resist. They resist because they're actually producers. They've just worked hard all their lives at whatever their specialty is. And they all kind of resist because they like doing what they do. They don't necessarily don't usually want to "go on disability." There's always kind of an internal hesitation about that."

Doctors Support

"We will look at medical records and help you determine if they're strong enough to go and make this claim. For example, if your doctors have been telling you for three years, you should stop working, right… Think about it from a doctor's perspective, "I'm trying to take care of you. You want me to fill out a disability form?" That is not their area of expertise. What patients need to understand is there's 20 different kinds of disability programs, right?

And they all mean something different. I'm getting that doctor again, not by telling them what to say, but how to say what they know is true and framing it within the confines of what are we looking for in a disability insurance policy. How can we make this real to the insurance company when someone presents with a symptom like brain fog or cognitive issues? How do we explain this as it is difficult to measure? We have different resources in the community that can do appropriate testing to measure some of these."

"Whether we're talking about syndrome like POTS or long-haul Covid, or even fibromyalgia and chronic fatigue, the most frustrating part of that for the patient journey is finding doctors who understand the disease process and believe the patient. A lot of doctors who don't understand the disease process won't believe the patient. It's not because the patient is lying, it's because the doctor just maybe doesn't have that experience. The hardest part of that journey and so many of our clients who come to us, they have been to one, two, three, or four doctors before they finally get referred to the one or the two who understand their illness and can help them. And then, as you know, it takes a long time. It can take a long time to get in to see the doctor and during Covid it took a longer time to get in to see these folks."

Medical Records
"Getting your own medical records and looking to see what the health care team is writing, is the first step. Check to

see is it accurate because sometimes even another person's records get mixed up with yours unfortunately. Because doctors are focused on getting you better and getting you to the next stage of your life, they're not often focused on documenting restrictions and limitations, documenting ways or reasons why this person can't work. Again. They're focused on the future. We can help by analyzing medical records and saying, you know, Christie, next time you see your doctor, you need to get her to assess you for ABC and to talk about ABC in the medical records."

Documentation

"My advice to people with chronic diseases is to document. For example, I may have a client who may have a migraine 17 days out of 30 in a month. We ask, "Are you keeping a migraine journal? Oh, no, I wasn't. Well, that's a really good idea." Or people will say, if I'm able to do one or two errands on Monday, but it really knocks me out until Wednesday. Okay, well, let's start at least journaling that. That really is for the claim, and also for your doctor. But really, we're helping to support the claim there."

Appealing Denials

"Having a lawyer look at a claim denial, figure out the exact reason why the insurance company is denying the claim, developing a strategic plan for filling those holes in it—sometimes it is different medical doctors, different testing, different medical records, sometimes its vocational services where you could learn about and transfer and do a different job. "

Long-Term Disability vs. Social Security Disability Insurance

Long-Term Disability (LTD) applies to a disability insurance policy that is either provided by an employer or purchased by an individual privately. Many companies, especially smaller employers, don't offer LTD insurance, and many people don't buy their own private policies. This is where government-supported SSDI in the US comes in as SSDI protects anyone who has worked long enough and recently enough to qualify.

One big difference between the two insurance programs is that LTD will normally protect you for a year or two (depending on the policy) if you are unable to work at your own occupation, even if you still have the capacity to work at a different occupation (for example, a surgical nurse who can no longer spend long hours standing but could work in a sedentary job at a nurse-staffed helpline). On the other hand, SSDI requires that you be unable to work at any job that meets their criteria (which vary by age). Both programs allow you to earn some money and still qualify for disability payments, if you are able.

Even if you have an LTD policy, you also will probably be applying for SSDI if you are unable to work at any job. That's because most LTD policies allow the insurance company to "offset" what they pay you for LTD benefits by what you receive from SSDI. Not applying for SSDI is not an option, because most policies allow the insurance company to offset even for what they say you would be "eligible to receive," even if you don't actually apply.

The medical community is seeing an alarming increase in POTS in patients recovering from Covid-19. The *Wall Street Journal* recently wrote about this unexpected increase in what has been a relatively rare condition. It's just one of a constellation of conditions that affect "Covid Long Haulers" or "Long Covid" people who have recovered from acute Covid-19 infection, but are dealing with lingering health conditions, such as POTS and chronic fatigue, that in some cases are disabling.

Ben Glass and his firm have substantial experience with POTS and disability claims, but he notes he doesn't yet know how the disability insurance industry will react to Covid-related "long-haul" claims for conditions such as POTS, However, based on experience, he thinks insurance companies seem to reserve special scrutiny for conditions that are not disabling for most people but may be disabling for a few. POTS fits squarely in that category. These suggestions also apply to other chronic illnesses.

Tips for applying for disability

Sometimes, it happens in an instant. Sometimes, it has been building for months or even years. Either way, the result is the same: You can no longer do your job. Now what?

How do I apply for LTD disability benefits?

With the disclaimer that every case is unique, here are some steps in common to nearly all claims for disability benefits:

1. Does your employer offer disability benefits? Some do, some don't. Employers are not required to offer disability insurance, but many do, especially larger employers. Call human resources to find out.

2. If the answer is no, your other option may be to apply for Social Security Disability Benefits.

3. If the answer is yes, your employer does offer disability benefits, ask for a copy of the policy and the summary plan description.

4. *Read policy documents carefully.* They should tell the specific steps you'll need to take to apply for disability benefits. Sometimes you work through human resources for employer's programs, but if an outside insurance company administers claims, you'll work with them directly.

5. The LTD policy documents will tell very important information, such as:

   - What makes you disabled (there will be a specific definition of "disabled" and "disability").

   - How long you need to be disabled before benefit payments start (this is usually called the Elimination Period).

   - How much your disability benefit is (it's normally a percentage of your salary; 60–80% is common).

   - What you need to provide to get benefits (called Proof of Claim).

- How to get started on your claim (often a phone call is all it takes, and then the insurance company will send you some forms to fill out as they determine whether or not to approve your claim).

6. The most important things to keep in mind:

- *You* have to provide proof of claim. The insurance company may help by requesting medical records for you, but ultimately it is *Your* responsibility to get them the forms they need from you and your doctor as well as your medical records.

- Talk to your doctor about your disability claim. There is no way around it: You have to have medical support to make a disability claim.

Application essentials

Documentation is essential. While POTS for example can be documented with objective tests, the impact of its symptoms (such as dizziness and fatigue) is largely subjective. If you suffer from POTS or hEDS and cannot do your job because of it, make sure your doctor understands and records what your symptoms are. We also recommend that you document your symptoms daily, share your symptom journal with your doctor, and make sure it becomes a part of your medical record. There are good online symptom-logging tools you can use, or you can keep a record in a journal (electronic or paper). At a minimum, be sure to note:

- Date;
- Symptoms you are experiencing that day;
- Severity (use whatever scale makes sense to you, but keep it consistent. Don't rate your dizziness a "6" on one day and "moderate" another day).
- Functional impact. What were you able to do/not do that day?

Be accurate with your journal. Surveillance and social media are being used to cross-check against your reported activity level at times. If your journal says you were in bed all day Monday, but surveillance shows you mowing your lawn, that's trouble. Better to log that you were in bed all morning, pushed yourself to mow the lawn for the first time in three weeks, had to take multiple breaks, and then spent the rest of the day in bed because you were exhausted from even that minimal activity. (Not-so-fun fact: some insurance companies are now using "unmanned surveillance," meaning they position small cameras in trees and on poles in your neighborhood and they come back to collect the footage later!)

Testing evidence is essential. There are tests for POTS, so to make a claim based on POTS you need to show the results of these tests, or your doctor needs to explain why they weren't indicated in your case. Disability reviewers will often look for:

- Tilt Table Test;
- EKG;
- EEG/QEEG;

- Nerve Conduction Study (EMG);
- Echocardiogram of heart and carotid arteries;
- Vascular studies;
- Bloodwork;
- Urinalysis;
- Ultrasound.

Some of these tests help diagnose POTS, while others help rule out other causes for your symptoms. All together, they show the disability reviewers that you and your doctor are trying to get an accurate diagnosis based on objective test results. This also is the case with any chronic illness: proper testing and medical documentation from your doctors to prove your diagnosis and symptoms.

Support from your doctor is essential. Your primary care doctor is a good place to start, but if your symptoms are so severe that they prevent you from working, it's best to get a referral to a doctor who specializes in your condition. Your doctor needs to explain to the insurance company or SSA through your office visit notes:

- Your diagnosis;
- The severity of your symptoms;
- Restrictions and limitations on your ability to function (these are what match your job duties to determine whether or not you can do your job);
- Your treatment plan;
- Your prognosis.

Bibliography

Reddy, Sumathi. "For Covid Long-Haulers, a Little-Known Diagnosis Offers Possible Treatments, and New Challenges." *The Wall Street Journal*, 30 November 2020, https://www.wsj.com/livecoverage/covid-2020-11-30/card/sTWuFEicwhllmmEaowqk.

ACKNOWLEDGMENTS

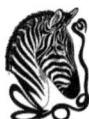

I've got a lot of people to thank who have helped along the way to develop this book

- *John S. Cox*
- *Hope Newton*
- *Inajo, John and Michael Cox*
- *Bill, Nancy, David, Veronica, Doug, Caroline and Lisa Hart, Mar Jo Lexa*
- *Eric Singman, MD*
- *Amanda Miller, PhD*
- *Sunil Patel, MD*
- *Chip Norris, PhD*
- *Cortney Gensemer, PhD*

- *Camille Schrier*
- *Trisha Torrey*

- *Wendy Quan*

- *Gwenn Herman*
- *Ellen Lenox Smith*
- *Ben Glass*
- *Beth Kallman Werner*
- *Olson Pook*

- *Hasan Abdallah, MD*
- *Annette Hudler, MD*

- *Alan Spanos, MD*
- *Lauren Stiles*
- *Lara Bloom*
- *Dorothy Poppe*
- *Cathy Poznik*
- *Momikai Jennings*
- *Jessica Beach*
- *Melissa Hale*
- *Elizabeth Shea*

- *Danielle Pool*
- *Avi Goldscheider*
- *Pam, Roman and Eden Fenner*
- *Kristin Means*
- *Cliona Molloy*
- *Paula Marolewski*
- *John Ferman*
- *Meghan Shaw*
- *Frani Mo*
- *Carrie Rein*
- *Matt Mailloux*
- *Phil Breddy*
- *Jana DiCarlo*

Thank you the patient community for contributing stories, responding to countless polls and sharing your artwork, including the unravelling zebra from 16-year-old Eden Fenner featured on each chapter intro and the poem from Cliona Molloy. I am eternally grateful for the gifts from you—my fellow patients, caregivers, medical providers seeking to learn and anyone giving the gift of understanding. If you've learned something helpful or enjoyed this book, please pay it forward by leaving an honest review or rate it by giving it an appropriate star if it guided you deeper in your journey to wellness! Every review matters, and it matters a lot because it might help someone else. Head over to Amazon or wherever you purchased this book to leave a review. All the zebras in the dazzle thank you endlessly.

INDEX